Incompatible with Nature

A Mother's Story

Tracie Frank Mayer

To Marc

"Nobody has ever measured, not even poets, how much the heart can hold."

~ Zelda Fitzgerald

Contents

Heart to Heart

Michael D. Freed, M.D.

While some of the vital organs are paired (lungs and kidneys) others are unitary (stomach liver, brain, etc.). While the heart seemingly is unitary, there are actually two sides of the heart that perform separate functions. There are two top chambers of the heart (atrium), two bottom chambers (ventricles) and two great arteries that leave the heart, the pulmonary artery and aorta. Blood with diminished oxygen and increased carbon dioxide from cellular metabolism travels via the systemic veins back to the heart and enters the right atrium, passes through a valve into the right ventricle and then is pumped out the pulmonary artery to the lungs. In the lungs the oxygen content is increased and the carbon dioxide content reduced. The blood then passes through the pulmonary veins into the left atrium, through a valve into the left ventricle, and then is pumped out into the aorta which carries blood enriched with oxygen to the various organs.*

While 99% of the time the heart develops normally in utero, approximately 1% of the time there is a problem usually involving one of the four heart valves, holes between the two atrium or ventricles or between the aorta and pulmonary artery or some combination of lesions. Although some problems are due to known chromosomal or gene abnormalities, the etiology of most are still unknown. Much less commonly, perhaps one in one hundred thousand, there seems to be a problem with the bilaterally and there is only one atrium, one ventricle or one vessel leaving the heart. When there are variations of venous return to the atrium there may be variations in the position of the abdominal organs and veins, usually called heterotaxy syndrome.

In Marc's case he had one of these heterotaxy syndromes with all the systemic veins coming back to the heart entering into a "common" atrium, a single large ventricle, and only one great vessel leaving the heart, in Marc's case the aorta. The pulmonary artery, the vessel going to the lungs was not connected to the heart. Until the 1970's these conditions were uniformly fatal, usually in the first few weeks or months of life.

In 1944 Drs. Blalock and Taussig suggested an operation to divert blood from one of the arteries that normally goes to the arm to the pulmonary artery but this was difficult to do, and with no "corrective" surgery was thought to be futile in this condition.

In 1971, Dr. Francis Fontan, a surgeon in Bordeaux France suggested an operation to divert blood from the veins directly into the pulmonary arteries, using the atrium, single ventricle and aorta to supply blood to the body. With modifications over the last 45 years this is the procedure that is now done in these circumstances and was done in Marc's situation. While not a corrective operation it has been found to be effective palliation that has allowed a near normal life for tens of thousands of children around the world.

*modified from:

http://www.heart.org/idc/groups/heart-public/@wcm/@hcm/documents/downloadable/ucm_307643.pdf

CHAPTER ONE

Something's Wrong

Marc had been relatively quiet lying upon the hard flat surface of the examination table, the two snaps on his undershirt open, exposing his tender stomach and tiny chest. I was thankful the small room was warm. Having positioned my chair as close to him as possible, I sat forward on its edge, and leaning over him, gently began stroking his head, his face, his left arm and leg, as it was the left side of his body that was closest to me. I would have gobbled him up completely if I'd known it wouldn't interrupt the examination. Comforting and reassuring him, I whispered my love to him.

"Everything's fine, sweetheart. Yes, yes, you are Mama's precious baby. You're being such a good boy, yes, darling. Mommy and Papa love you. Everything's fine, everything's fine. Mama's sweetie thing."

His precious mutterings fluttered like colorful butterflies in the air. Occasionally he would wiggle or thrust his tiny legs. All the while I stroked and kissed and patted him, completely enthralled. Every time I looked at him I was overwhelmed by that "I can't believe my baby is here in front of my eyes and I love him so much I can't stand it!" feeling. My heart and soul burned with intense devotion to him. Watching him turn his head from time to time, I could swear he looked as if he were observing the world around him, perhaps curious about the intruder zigzagging across his chest. Thirteen days old. I wondered how large his thoughts were.

His almond eyes widened when he turned his head towards my voice, his tiny rosebud mouth open, searching for my index finger that caressed his cheek. Having become so personally acquainted with him the last thirteen days, I was well aware of his strong sucking instinct. I recalled the picture safely tucked away of him taken at twelve weeks: an ultrasound image of him floating on his back, feet in the air, his thumb in his mouth.

I had already decided before his birth that I would not use a *Schnuller* as a magic wand to instantly quiet his cries, or encourage his contentment. I was there for him. What on earth would he need a pacifier for? My finger, at the ready, was bent into position; it would be the smooth arch of the crook of that finger that he would welcome into his mouth. I knew that he wasn't yet hungry, and was sure that this appeasement would help to allay any discomfort. It pleased me: mother, satisfier. Inundated with an overwhelming rush of love, I had more than a desire to nurture, protect and provide for him; I wanted to be his everything.

Though completely new to babies and their needs, I wasn't at all nervous, in fact I felt at home with being my son's mother. Besides the fact that God had blessed me with child, I found further reward in the absolute joy I felt when my baby was at peace, sated and content. Funny what we find gratifying at different stages of our lives.

From the moment the Professor opened his undershirt and squirted a gel on his tiny chest and began carefully sliding the scanner of the ultrasound machine back and forth in the gooey mass, he had neither fretted nor fussed. And he never cried. He mesmerized me.

Helmut sat to the left of me, his hand on my lap, his fingers every now and again lightly tapping. His touch reassured me, just as his touching me reassured him, just as I was sure my touch reassured Marc. My husband's hand on me, my hand on our son; a chain linked by touch, by love.

We looked attentively at the scanner sliding slowly back and forth, observed it making its way under each side of our son's neck, inching toward his chest, hesitating on the left side, then the right. It slid down toward his stomach, pausing. Up again toward his chest. Left, then right. Back and forth. Up and down. Side to side. Slowly.

The images on the monitor that the scanner produced told us nothing. It might as well have been Greek. Helmut covered my left fist with his right hand and pulled it to the folds of his lap. He held it a few moments there, tight and still. I don't know if it was the throbbing of his pulse that I felt or mine. Soon I was aware of him unpeeling my clammy fingers and opening my hand, pressing it flat against his pant leg. He squeezed it for but a moment, patted it twice, then crowned it with his palm.

The squeeze and the pats implied that even if he were to remove his hand, I was not to remove mine. Though I couldn't speak German and he struggled with English, we had our own language; a certain touch, look or movement spoke volumes that only we understood. I glanced at the side of his face. It immediately revealed the tension that was gnawing at the both of us.

Prior to our marriage six months earlier, that time when we each lived on different continents, the very thought of him would quicken my pulse. And in my mind's eye, his eyes and his lips, indeed his very spirit was always smiling. His lips were now an incision in a face rigid and sober. His upper jaw jutted in and out as if he were clenching his teeth. Clenching and releasing. Clenching and releasing. I had never seen him this way and I didn't like it. I began squirming in my seat. Why was this taking so long?

I looked expectantly at the Professor. Sitting on the opposite side of the examination table, he was within reach.

"Is this your first baby? So what brought you all the way to Germany from America? Oh, I see! Now that is true love. How long have you lived here now? Um-hmm... Well, I speak a bit of English, but I prefer of course to speak German... Is there a big difference living here compared with living in America? Which city do you come from? It is a beautiful day today, isn't it? Don't worry. The examination won't hurt your son."

Small talk that happened only in my mind. His sharply chiseled profile never cracked to emit a sound, not even a goo-goo gaga to our son. Too hard-boiled to even clear his throat, he stayed the course, continuously gliding the scanner. Removing his eyes from the monitor only long enough to check his hand position, his gaze remained fixed on the screen.

I wanted to reach out and tap him on the shoulder and ask, "Doctor, so what is it exactly that you're looking for? How many times have you done this? Why is it taking so long? Why haven't we been told by somebody, by – ANYBODY – why we're here? Do all new born babies here in Germany get this examination or is this an international procedure? Is this the last stop? What is that little dot pulsating there?" But I didn't dare. He had an impenetrable aura. Reserved. Cool as granite. Maybe it was his title that stopped me in my tracks; maybe one shouldn't speak with the Professor unless spoken to. Perhaps it was his crisp white doctor's coat. Out of nowhere the question of etiquette between doctor and patient popped into my mind. Is there such a thing I wondered? How does it work? Should my questions wait until the end of the exam, would it be rude to ask for an explanation during? Would it irritate? Make him angry? And then there was the language matter. I didn't know if he understood English and if he didn't, the resulting chopped up English and disjointed German "did I understand him" – "did she understand me" – "did I understand her" – "and he me" problem was not worth the headache. I wasn't up to Germanic aerobics. "Just let him get on with it," I told myself. "In a little while this will all be over. He's going to tell you everything's fine anyway – so just let him have his peace so he can hurry up and get finished and we can pack up and get out of here." He never comforted me, never told me to relax, so I didn't. I couldn't. You see, in the back of my mind, I kept thinking, if someone is sent to a hospital he or she is sent there for a reason, but I had no clue as to why we'd been sent here. And I was absolutely certain everything was fine with our baby. So what was going on? Jesus. There were no cushions to adjust on this uncomfortable chair.

Thirty minutes had passed; a journey from the cradle to the grave. No one had said a word and I was growing wearier by the minute. Aside from Marc's sweet murmurs and my whispers, an eerie, uncomfortable silence pervaded the room. It provided no indication of the volcano about to erupt. He continued to guide the scanner. Then, with his eyes still fixed on the monitor, his German accent thick and heavy, the Professor finally uttered, *"Was ich sehe ist leider nicht gut."*

Smacking his palm to his forehead, his face twisted in pain, Helmut released an anguished sigh and slumped back in his chair. I stiffened ramrod straight in mine. An undefined feeling of fear gripped me with such force I could barely breathe. Without thinking, I snatched a fistful of Helmut's jacket sleeve with one hand while my other clutched at Marc. My voice suddenly hoarse, as if my vocal chords had been seared, I could at first only muster a whisper.

"What did he say, Helmut?"

Though it was only a moment, it seemed a lifetime before he answered me. From where he was sitting, he could not really see the Professor's face. I could. Leaning slightly to the right and stretching my neck to look over his shoulder, I could see that his face revealed nothing other than a stable equilibrium. A moment...Perhaps he was waiting for the Professor to say that he'd erred, that we could in fact breathe again. Perhaps he just didn't believe his ears or thought he had misunderstood him. The Professor continued sliding the scanner.

Grating my chair against the floor, I released Helmut's arm and grabbed his shoulder as I jumped to my feet, the chain still linked to our son. I panicked as I tried to blink away the blinding flashes of light that distorted my vision. The walls were closing in. I had to stay calm. This would all be cleared up. Trapped in a sudden heat of terror that ripped at my gut and weakened my bowels, I couldn't have screamed if I wanted to. The dampness rising in my armpits assured me that a war was about to erupt in the heavens and it would be out of my control. I was defenseless against the "*Was ich sehe ist leider nicht gut*" ringing in my ears.

I didn't understand the words but Helmut's outburst destabilized me. Scared me senseless. I could hear myself trying to breathe. I nearly tore off the leather skin of the jacket at his shoulder. Trying to keep myself under control my voice broke.

"What did he say, Helmut?"

I sensed the Professor's eyes on me.

"*Spricht Ihre Frau Deutsch?*" ("Does your wife speak German?")

Helmut shook his head. "No," he said.

With his hand still to his forehead, his elbow now supported by the examination table, Helmut raised his free hand and groped for mine. He turned and looked up at me, tears brimmed his eyes. He winced before he spoke and when he finally did, his voice sounded as if it belonged to someone else.

"Something's wrong," he whispered.

CHAPTER TWO

Just a Checkup

We arrived promptly at the Children's Department of Cardiology at the University Clinic of Cologne for our eleven A.M. appointment. It was Thursday, the 13th of December, 1984.

The sliding glass doors at the main entrance automatically opened as we stood before them. Once inside, Helmut led us towards a sign that said *Anmeldung*. He greeted the woman behind the glass window of the registration desk. Feeling inside the left breast pocket of his jacket, he pulled out the scheduled appointment paper we'd been issued from Weyerthal, the hospital where our son crossed that threshold from my pelvis to my arms. She glanced at the document then directed us to the first floor.

Helmut held one side of Marc's carry-cot while I held the other as we made our way up the stairs to the first landing. From the moment we first lost ourselves in each other, our rhythm was always in sync; even ascending the staircase the balls of our feet scraped each step in unison; right left right left right left right. A few feet away from the top of the landing was a door with big black blocked letters: *KINDER KARDIOLOGIE ABTEILUNG* (Children's Cardiology Department). Helmut pushed the door open. We found ourselves in a well-lit waiting room. He placed his strap of the carry-cot in my hand.

"You and Marc get a seat, sweetie. I'll go let the secretary know we are here.

Because I couldn't speak German, I didn't want to be bothered with someone speaking to me, then having to concentrate, and with a little bit of guesswork figuring out what I thought they had said and in a split second, so as to not look a fool, determine what or how I would answer; if I'd smile and nod my head and *"Ja"* them or frown and shake my head and *"Nein"* them, or grin and *"Schön"* them depending on their facial expressions. No. I was not up to the strain of it. Not now. I headed toward an unoccupied corner of the room.

I kissed Marc and cradled him gently. Then, just in case a draft should find its way into the room, I reached over into his cot and removed a lightweight rainbow-colored blanket my Aunt Audrey had crocheted for him and draped it over his waist and legs. It was light enough not to be burdensome and yet provided just that right amount of cover. Its cheeriness contrasted sharply with the gloom that drifted throughout the waiting room.

Uneasiness began to envelope me. What on earth were we doing here? Slowly, the smell of a chemical agent began to invade my nostrils and penetrate the surface of my skin. After the first couple of moments, I guessed what it could be: a confusing potpourri of disinfectant mixed with buttered *Brötchen* (bread rolls), coffee, rubbing alcohol and sterilized needles. A frightening but somehow suitable smell for this room, for this place.

And though the lofty, whitish walls were sporadically splotched with pictures drawn by children, it didn't feel like a kid-friendly place. Poster-sized announcements of upcoming events at the hospital decorated the room. My stomach began to flutter each time I inhaled. Aside from the recovery time after giving birth to our son, I'd never been in a hospital in my life and had absolutely no idea what to expect. Helmut, having completed our registration, was closing the door behind him and heading straight towards us. Thank goodness.

"Is this normal, Helmut? I mean, is this what all parents do when they get kids in Germany?"

At first, I didn't earnestly pay attention to his answer; I knew he didn't know anyway. I just needed to ask, to say something to make a verbal connection, break the nervous tension. My attention had been drawn to two older children entertaining themselves at a wooden play table in the middle of the room. They occupied themselves with the few books and toys scattered about, and it wasn't long after I'd sat down that their constant chatter, sporadic outbursts and the scraping of their chairs against the floor began to grate on my brittle nerves.

More disturbing, their parents did nothing to quiet them. "What is wrong with these people? Why don't they make their kids quiet down? I will never let my child carry on like that. They're big enough to know how to behave in a public place, even if they are at the kids' table."

"Calm down," I told myself. "Calm down. Calm. Down. You're just nervous because you don't know what's going on. You don't understand it whatever it is. This is surely just the routine checkup you get when you have a baby. They probably do this all over the world for all I know. It's not helping that Helmut doesn't know why the station doctor from Weyerthal Hospital sent us here either - though he should - it's his country, damn it!" Lost in thought, I didn't recognize that he'd twisted in his seat so he could comfortably put his arm around me. Squeezing my shoulder, he answered me.

"I don't know, sweetie, I never had a baby before," he smiled. "But don't worry, I'm sure everything's fine. If something was wrong, someone would have told us by now. Don't forget, you stayed twelve days in the hospital with him and you had all your checkups from your doctor before he was born and everything was fine. Don't worry, sweetie."

Nodding, I corroborated this by counting Marc's fingers and toes as I cuddled him. He looks fine, I thought. I don't know anything about babies, but he looks fine. Helmut's right. If something was wrong, surely we'd know it by now. I tried to relax.

Did my level best.

"We've scheduled you an appointment at the University Clinic's Children's Cardiology Department. It's just a checkup," I remembered the attending nurse saying as we were about to check out of the room Marc and I had occupied since his birth nearly two weeks before. It seemed like an inordinately long time, but it was normal at the time for women to stay so long in the hospital after a caesarean section at this particular hospital. She handed Helmut the document with the scheduled appointment. I flew to his side and examined the document; deciphering *Kinder, Kardiologie* and *Universitäts Klinik* and my child's name was not difficult.

"No need to be alarmed. It's just a checkup," Helmut said the nurse said.

White haired and matronly, past her prime and comfortable with that, perhaps she was an Oma, she seemed the grandmotherly type. Immediately sensing my alarm at the mention of clinic and cardiology, she wasted no time in comforting me. I played her words over and over again in my mind. "It's just a checkup," she said, patting my arm. With her smiling eyes and gentle voice, she was reassuring.

We were in that hospital for twelve days, I thought, trying logically to calm myself down. If something was not in order somebody surely would have said something by now. Wouldn't they have? My obstetrician-gynecologist checked us regularly. I had a printout of our baby's fetal heart rate made when I was three months pregnant. Everything was fine. And the snapshot of him taken at twelve weeks from the sonogram where he was sucking his thumb; everything was as it should be. Come on, kiddo, you've never been a needless worrier. You have no reason to entertain the notion that something is not in order. I looked to Helmut. He kissed my cheek and wrapped our son's tiny hand around his little finger. We were quiet for a time, each nursing our own thoughts. I crossed my right leg over my left. Couldn't stop it from twitching.

Helmut, not a sit still and do nothing type, immersed himself in a magazine while I repeatedly stole glances into the faces of the other parents. I didn't want to invade their unsheltered space. You couldn't help but look at them and wonder which shadow had intercepted the light in their lives and landed them here.

I said a silent prayer that their babies were fine, but I also prayed to God that if one of these babies had a problem, let it not be mine. Everybody looked so grim, as if the weight of the world had been dropped on their shoulders. Was I reading resignation on their blank faces? I mean, they were here just like us, probably first visit and all, just dotting the i's and crossing the t's, right? How could they be resigned to the boogeyman if they didn't even know he existed?

On the right side of the room, closest to the door with the big blocked letters, sat a Turkish couple. Several times the man stood and paced the room. She remained seated, her abundant hips providing their baby ample cushion to lie across her lap; legs parted, crossed at the ankle. Her right hand rested on the child's back as she rocked him. Other than myself, they were the only foreigners in the room.

Occupying two chairs along the opposite wall a young couple sat silently side by side; she holding their baby in her arms, he sitting forward on his chair; his blond head bowed, hands clasped and hanging between bent knees. Neither of them seemed to be affected by the laughter and clatter emanating from the kids at the table. Particularly amazing because one of the kids belonged to them. I felt their eyes on me as we entered the room. I looked over at them. They quickly looked away.

Several chairs' distance away from me, a grandmother spoke quietly to her daughter, sometimes cooing and making animated faces to the grandbaby her daughter cradled. She and her daughter ignored her older grandchild, the other youngster making so much noise at the play table in the middle of the room. The strain was palpable.

Marc slept peacefully in my arms. Other than the door to the secretary's office, there were two other doors adjacent to this room; to the right of the secretary's office was the entrance door, to the left the other door which occasionally opened, smacking the air each time it did. Its glass window was murky and I couldn't help but wonder what was happening on the other side. Before it shut, that strange smell was always stronger in the waiting room.

Several times nurses and doctors hurriedly bustled through with files and folders in hand. Other than getting a bit tripped up when they spotted me, they never fell out of step. They could have at least nodded or smiled or done something to alleviate the seriousness in there. When the door smacked the air again, a nurse called us in. I didn't hear it shut behind us, but sometimes doors close without making a sound.

We faced a corridor. A row of connecting chairs lined a portion of the wall at its far end. That smell hung heavy in the air now. Several rooms were located along this long hallway; we were shown into an examination room on the left just a few steps away from the smacking door. The room was not very big and though the curtains were closed, the lights were on, so at least it wasn't dark.

Three adult-sized chairs framed an ultrasound machine and the examination table; one chair purposefully placed next to the equipment on one side of the table by itself, the other two on the opposite side, next to each other. Two extra chairs stood against a wall, and nearby was a small washbasin. An overhead mirror hung above it. Several small white cabinets hung suspended from two walls, a larger one rooted to the floor.

We sat in the two chairs next to each other. It was warm, almost stuffy in this dull room. Shortly after we settled ourselves, we heard two faint knocks on the door and it opened. Helmut stood as the doctor entered the room.

"Good day, Professor. I am Helmut Mayer." He and the Professor clasped hands for a moment, then Helmut turned to me.

"This is my wife, and this is our son, Marc."

"*Guten Tag*," he nodded, not quite smiling at me and offering his hand.

Not wanting to disturb Marc, I extended my hand from underneath my precious bundle as far as it would go. He walked over to me and accepted what little he could of my fingertips. I took careful inventory of his features. The first thing I noticed was his hair. Thick and straight and black as coal. The thickness naturally parted on the side, scissors had forced it all into a respectable cut, trimmed above the ears and collar. Sea-blue eyes set in a chiseled face. A serious face without laugh lines. And he had delicate hands.

"*Guten Tag.*" I smiled up at him.

He nodded again. Without further ado, he took his seat opposite us within reach of the diagnostic equipment of the ultrasound machine. He opened the file that he'd brought into the room with him, briefly scanned the top sheet, then instructed me, but addressing Helmut in German, to remove Marc's clothing so that his upper body was exposed.

He then said to place him on the examination table. I left his undershirt on. Because it had snaps on either side, I figured it could be opened right before the examination started and then quickly closed when finished.

The examination table was concealed by a crisp cotton white sheet. I covered the area where our son would be lying with one of our blankets and then as though I was holding a rare, priceless object of art, I carefully laid him atop, easing his little jumpsuit down to the beginnings of his diaper, leaving his legs and feet inside.

This was after all just a checkup and we'd surely be out of here sooner rather than later. It wasn't necessary to make him uncomfortable by completely undressing him.

Any Moment

I didn't realize I had collapsed into my chair. Though Helmut was right next to me, close enough to comfortably hug me, I strained to see his face clearly. And when I could, I looked at him as I had never done before. He must have lost his mind. My breath was coming to me in little hitches, the flat of my left hand pressed against the heaving of my chest.

"What do you mean something's wrong, Helmut?"

The Professor addressed me, his face wooden, his English unsteady.

"The baby is very sick. You must leave him here. We must watch him tonight. Tomorrow I will make more tests."

My eyes drifted away from his face and lingered upon our son, my angel child, the manifestation of true love, of my womb, Helmut's and my everything...He must be kidding. My eyes locked with his. It was like looking down the barrel of a gun.

"What? What are you talking about? What do you mean leave our baby here? Why? What's the matter with him? No! No! For what? I'm NOT leaving my baby here! Helmut! Helmut, tell him we are not leaving Marc here! He's not sick! There can't be something wrong! Nobody ever EVER said anything about him being sick, Helmut. His checkups were always fine! You know it! Tell him! Tell him to call the obstetrician! Tell—"

"The baby is so ill he could die at any moment," the Professor cut me off.

His words reverberated like ricochets around the room.

I froze. Time stood perfectly still. Staring blankly into his face I could feel myself helplessly falling through space, slowly, ever so slowly toppling into an abyss. My – baby – is – so – ill – he – could die? At any moment? I looked at his face in utter disbelief, dumbfounded. I felt faint. And for the very first time that I could ever remember, I was speechless. The room fell silent. Then I burst out crying, and stepped over the edge.

I don't remember the details of the ensuing melee. The door to the examination room had been inadvertently left ajar. But when? I was sure the Professor closed it after he first came in. Pacing. Everyone was pacing. The Professor had left the room for a moment and had come back with a nurse, they were both whispering, walking back and forth in front of me. Helmut, too, around the examination table, back and forth, pacing. Nurses, doctors and parents all were keeping up the tempo outside the door to our room unashamedly peeking inside at me as they walked past, curious to see the source of the commotion, a hysterical woman in a state of delirium.

Only Marc and I remained glued to our designated places, the both of us helpless. Where was everybody going? The absolute destruction of the unnatural silence in the corridor must have relieved the other parents waiting there. For whatever problems they may have had, they were surely not as bad as the problem in the examination room at the end of the hall by the smacking door where that poor lady was screaming and crying. My wails must have reassured them. Comforted them that they weren't alone in their woes.

The nurse who had accompanied the Professor into the room was trying to explain to me in her native tongue, with sympathetic eyes and a finger pointing towards the door that she had to take our baby to another room. By now, several of the staff had entered the room. They all tried to calm me down, to no avail. Their mouths were soft pliable holes that simply moved in their faces. Babel assaulted my senses when they spoke. Even if I would have understood their language, I wouldn't have understood what they were saying anyway.

I knew I'd parked the car, turned off the ignition, but it was still rolling. Pumping the brakes did not bring it to a halt. I remember watching the nurse with the kind eyes wipe the gooey gel off of our son's chest and dress him, then gently lift him into her arms, turn and then disappear from the room. As if jabbering and pointing towards the door presumed my permission to take my child from me. It took a moment for me to register that she had actually left the room with him. I jumped up after her, Helmut on my heels, the Professor behind him. We landed in the opposite end of the corridor past more rooms and the nurses' station, in front of a row of connecting chairs.

I was confused...dazed...lost. Couldn't focus through my tears, couldn't figure out where I was, or which way to turn. God in Heaven. Where was my baby? Another nurse suddenly appeared before me carrying a glass of water in one hand, a pill in the other. The Professor had instructed her to give me a tranquilizer. I looked at her as if she were stupid.

"I DON'T WANT A GODDAMNED TRANQUIL-IZER! I'M BREASTFEEDING MY BABY!"

My nose was running and I could feel myself screaming, but did they hear me? Didn't they get it? Didn't all these highly trained medical professionals understand that a woman breastfeeding her child wasn't going to take a goddamned tranquilizer? Did I have to spell it out?

"Where's my baby?!" I dismissed the tranquilizer with an impatient wave of my hand. The nurse said something and raised her arms a little higher, trying once again to make me accept her offering. This is really not her fault, I managed to tell myself. She's just trying to carry out her orders. She has really no idea that you have absolutely no intention of swallowing that pill, and that if she doesn't hurry up and tell you where the hell your baby is you just might shove it down her throat.

"Your baby's fine."

I spun around. English! English! Thank you God, I sobbed. I'd been saved. Saved! I suddenly had a rope to cling to. He could speak my language. Fluently. His hospital whites told me he was a doctor. He could help me. I knew it.

"Where's my baby?"

Dr. Gillor had been summoned by Susannah, one of the nurses of this ward.

"There's a new patient," she told him. "The mother is from America. The Professor needs you. You can speak English."

Somehow, I ended up in one of the rooms off the corridor with him. We sat facing each other. My face was no longer my own; tears and snot, shock and fear masked me.

"What's your name?" he asked me.

"Tracie."

He looked at me and could barely conceal a kind smile.

"Not your first name. Your family name."

"Mayer."

I pronounced my new last name without a trace of my American accent. Mayer. One of the most common of German names, that is the last name he expected to hear tumbling from my lips as he sat there looking at me. The pieces of the puzzle didn't fit for him. There I was: brown skin, long black hair, twenty-eight years old, and in his eyes dressed *ausgefallen* – differently. In my mind, one man's sartorial splendor is another man's favorite pair of jeans. I don't remember what I wore that tumultuous day. He says I glittered. He told me later that they weren't used to the likes of me. Said I looked like a pop star. Sure. With my face splotched, tear-smeared. Black eyeliner and mascara streaked the area from my eyes to my chin like burned rubber marks from ill-fated auto-mobile tires.

"There is a problem with the baby's heart," he tried to make me understand, crossing his legs and leaning forward on his chair.

My outbursts had quieted down. I had come to the realization that no matter how much I screamed and cried, these people, these doctors, could not all be fools. My hysterics could not change the prognosis. Overcome by shock, I struggled to stay inside my skin. If I breathed deeply and slowly, perhaps I could stop the room from spinning. Concentrate. I had to try and get a grip on myself. There was something extremely serious going on here concerning our baby, and for him, if for no other reason, I had to pull myself together. Now.

"And it appears to be very serious," Dr. Gillor said.

I stumbled.

"What appears to be very serious?" I said.

"The situation with the baby's heart."

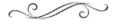

I couldn't yet focus, having just come from the room where the nurse had taken our son. It was just to the left of the long row of connecting chairs: the infant and small children's cardiology ward. Babies, nurses' station, medicines, disinfectant. The potpourri hanging in the air. The door was open. I was on my way into the room when I was distracted by a nurse. Before we could enter, she instructed Helmut and me to don green cotton sterilized hospital gowns over our clothes. I saw our son before I slipped into mine.

Standing on my toes in the doorway, leaning onto its frame for support, I craned my neck looking past the maze of cribs, machines, tables and chairs and adults staring at me. I wiped my tearstained eyes and runny nose on the back of my hand, squinted, and over there to the left, on the far side of the room I saw him being cradled in the arms of a nurse and sucking...a bottle. I felt a twitch in my leaking breasts. It's not important now, I told myself. At least he's eating and she's being careful with him.

I hurriedly got into the gown. Helmut was still fumbling with the snaps on my back as we entered the room. Marc's clothes had been removed. He was now wearing another undershirt and a white cotton knit long-armed top underneath a yellow velour cotton jumpsuit. Across the top of the little knit top and the jumpsuit were the words *Universitäts Kliniken Köln* (University Clinics Cologne). I did not believe this.

It seemed that just moments ago we were on our way here and Helmut was saying that as soon as the checkup was over, we would stop in one of the charming confectionary houses and luxuriate over a cup or two of smooth-flavored coffee and indulge in a good-to-the-last-bite slice of freshly baked cake. Maybe even two slices. The three of us would kiss and hug and cuddle in the midst of gingerbread houses, porcelain tableware and a treasury of traditional cookies synonymous with the holiday season in this country. Cheerful waitresses and cordial patrons would smile their congratulations at us. And I would be downright giddy with glee knowing that without a doubt this would be the most wonderful Christmas of my life.

How had I gone from that, the promise of cake and coffee and the most blessed time of my life not even an hour ago, to this ward with its strange smelling potpourri wafting in the air and this sterilized green gown and a nurse feeding my thirteen-day-old baby who could 'die at any moment'? What happened?

She smiled up at Helmut and me. Did I smile back? I don't know. I wanted to thank her for being gentle with our son and say, "Please don't forget to burp him - he likes it the most when you run your hand up and down his back while you gently pat him, remember to wipe his mouth and since you're there you might as well wipe his entire face, and please warm the lotion in your hands before you apply it to his face and neck and please don't let him keep a wet diaper on too long and make sure after you've changed him to clean his bottom with a baby wipe and then with a warm soapy washcloth and don't forget to smear the baby cream all over his bottom and top that off with a puff of powder before you put the fresh diaper on, and no he doesn't need a pacifier and..."

Instead I looked around the room. Life-sized rectangular windows behind the cribs ran the entire length of the wall and welcomed rays of ample sunlight. The upper half of the wall on the right side of the room by the entry was actually a big double window, blue curtains slashed back on either side. White cabinets lined all the walls and every inch of available floor space in that room. There were probably ten cribs in there, safety slats all pulled up.

Peep. Peep. Peep. Peep. Peep. Peep. Shrill, though not painfully loud, a note of warning pierced the room at regular intervals. Though several adults were talking in the room, and babies occasionally cried, I could only hear this constant steady ting-a-ling alarm. My swollen eyes drifted from wall to ceiling and from crib to crib until I figured it out: electrocardiogram monitors stationed by each bed were the cause. With each peep, a penny- sized heart with a number next to it blinked on the upper right corner of the screen. But how?

I looked closely at our son still in the arms of the nurse. His chest. I thought it looked somewhat lumpy when I first saw him. And then I saw the long beige cables sinuously making a path from the back of his little jumpsuit towards the monitor by his crib. Several strips of adhesive covered the gauze which secured the needle in his tiny wrist: medication via intravenous infusion. I was confused beyond comprehension.

Sitting within the confines of the consultation room, I tried to give my mind to what Dr. Gillor was saying to me. Only problem was, it didn't make one iota of sense. Not in English. Not in German. Not in Swahili. Not at all. Period. You can pistol-whip the fates later, I told myself. Now you must pay attention pay attention pay attention.

You know, it's the strangest feeling trying to hold on when there's nothing to hold on to. Over the edge, you're so far out there that you know veering round is not an option. So you start groping because you can't see. Reaching out, taking timid steps, afraid to move but knowing you must, you only grab a hold of nothingness in a fog so thick you can cut it with a knife, but you keep reaching, sure that you will come upon a tree or a wall or a shoulder or something to help you find your bearings. But there is...nothing.

It's a sensation that I imagine akin to the seconds before drowning and desperately trying to come up for air, but no matter how fiercely you fight the torrents, you remain submerged in a fury of impotence until you finally succumb and let go and you slip away into the depths of unawareness because you have no compass, you are un-engined; there...is...nothing...you...can do.

In letting go, you let the monster devour you. But for some reason, somewhere, somewhere deep, deep inside, you still feel a flicker of hope; maybe it's the wishful thinking that the monster doesn't devour you in one gulp, but it's hope nonetheless. Hope revolving around futility. The blessing and the curse of it all.

"So...um, what appears to be so serious about it?" I said.

"From the ultrasound examination the Professor made, there appear to be some serious anomalies."

"Uh-huh." I blew and wiped my nose. "What are anomalies?"

"Irregularities. Abnormalities."

"Oh...like what?"

"Well, instead of four chambers to the heart, it appears that he has only two."

"Um-hmm. Two...I see." I didn't see anything.

"But we'll know tomorrow after the heart catheterization," he said.

"Uh-huh."

His words hung in the air for a time while I tried to weigh their meaning. I had no idea what he was talking about.

"Heart catheterization," I repeated.

Helmut and the Professor entered the room sometime around that point. We'd somehow become separated between the ward and me finding my way into this chair. Seeing him did not snap me out of my zombie-like state. He looked as wretched as I did. He plopped into the chair next to me, pulled my hand to his lap and sadly sighed over and again. A nurse brought in Marc's empty carry-cot.

My heart skipped a beat and I was distinctly aware of a tightening in my stomach. The Professor picked up where Doctor Gillor left off. Half English. Half German. After carrying out the catheterization tomorrow, he would be able to tell us more. We should go home and try to get some rest. We could call him tonight at eight o'clock to see if there were any changes.

We looked in on Marc before we left. A wave of relief washed over me to see no apparent sign of distress in his unconsciousness; he was in a deep peaceful sleep. This, despite the medicine flowing through the tube intravenously in his arm, the high-pitched tone of the monitors and the cables snaking out from underneath his clothes. Thank God all this didn't seem to dramatically disturb him. It nearly killed me. Looking down at my flesh and blood lying there in that crib I did not believe my eyes.

"Could die at any moment." I flinched each time the Professor's words hammered in my ears. He can't be serious! I couldn't grasp the reality of the situation. I gripped the slats of the crib, trying to bend the metal until my fingertips hurt. My heart had been broken, but maybe if I could hurt myself externally, somewhere that I could see it, maybe break my fingers or begin to bleed, this moment would become real for me.

My eyes drifted down to the floor. Reflexively, I stomped on it a couple of times and was keenly aware of the fact that it didn't move. Okay, I thought. Okay. Hanging on to the slats of the crib with my right hand, I steadied myself into an upright position and raised the palm of my left hand and held it before my face. Beneath a furrowed brow my eyes followed the contour. I then slowly turned my hand around as if seeing it for the first time and observed the oval-shaped tips of red nails extending over the end of my fingers. Yes, this is your hand. You're making progress, I told myself. You recognize your own hand and the floor is not moving. You are here, instead of not here. This is real.

I lowered my hand so that I could grip the slats with both hands again and peered through them at our son. My heart lurched and I needed to swallow and breathe at the same time. I turned away so that my choking wouldn't wake him. Helmut gently patted my back.

"Are you okay, sweetie?"

"Yes, I'm...I'm fine."

And in that moment before I turned back towards our son, standing there struggling to shake off the disbelief and draw an even breath, I was overcome by such a swell of harrowing emotion that I didn't give a damn about the babies, the nurses, the parents, or the doctors. I just wanted to scream that it was simply not possible that the fates could so suddenly, so unexpectedly, and so mercilessly attack. Just not possible! Not by any stretch of the imagination! For a split second I thought it was too late. It took every bit of self-restraint not to let go.

Helmut left my side for a few moments. He'd gone to ask the nurse who had taken care of Marc to keep an eye out on him, and when she left her shift, to please ask her colleague to do the same. She promised she would. I had lowered the slats and was lightly drifting a finger over Marc's fingers. Helmut had returned. We kissed our son again and again. I quietly lifted the slat. Helmut took my hand in his. With the other he picked up the carry-cot and carried it in one hand to the car. The weight must have been unbearable.

Outside, the skies threatened. Though it was very late in the afternoon, almost evening, it wasn't the serene twilight of dusk that would be easing into a peaceful nightfall. I was quite sure the sun was shining when we got there. Sunless, moonless, starless, the atmosphere had changed to accommodate the absolute fracturing of my spirit. Of our spirits. We dragged each other to the car, clinging to one another in utter and profound devastation.

We drove to Maytex, a floor-covering store Helmut opened two years before. It was the closest place where we could stop and make a phone call. We had no cell phones then. Home was another few blocks away. Searching for an explanation, the first call was to my obstetrician/gynecologist; it was brief. Helmut spoke with him. What did he say? I don't really know... Maybe I don't remember. I guess it wasn't important. After all, what could he do? Yes, of course, he was shocked ... Yes, of course.

The next call Helmut made was to our insurance company. He'd had the very good sense to insure Marc right at his birth, so his medical care was covered. Thank God.

Then we called my family in Seattle, Washington. Helmut dialed the number. Since we'd been given the devastating news, my uncontrollable quivering had never stopped and breathing came to me in pants or deep sighs. I was like a marionette with strings attached to my limbs that were being manipulated by demented demons. Daddy answered the phone. When I heard his voice, the dam broke releasing my sobs. Again.

"Daddy," I wailed, "Something's wrong with Marc!"

He didn't say anything to me. Instead, he yelled over the receiver, "One of you better pick up the phone! Something's wrong with the baby!" Daddy's cry spread panic like a wildfire in the house. In seconds my mother and my two sisters picked up the telephone extensions. Though Mama and Daddy had come to Germany and stayed a few days for Marc's birth, I hadn't seen my sisters since I'd left home seven months before.

"Tracie! What's the matter?!"

They didn't believe me.

And then Helmut and I drove home. We called the hospital every hour or so until the wee hours of the morning. Marc was fine. Eating, sleeping.

"Herr Mayer, you and your wife should get some rest."

Um-hmm. Right. I didn't think I'd ever rest again. Ever.

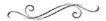

I stood in Marc's room that night. Looked around at all the furnishings, the toys, the stuffed animals, all the happiness and welcomeness that had greeted his homecoming the day before. With the smell of baby powder and lotion hanging in the air, his empty crib looked so odd, the room so silent. Without him, everything was out of place. Home sweet home cancelled.

I wrapped my arms around my stomach. A sense of hollowness engulfed me and there was absolutely nothing to fill the void. I knew I'd been pregnant. Knew I really had given birth to my precious child. I wasn't dreaming that I was in this house, in this city, in this country, married.

I fell to my knees by his crib and begged God to help me and to take care of our child, to lift this burden of grief that was slowly killing me, to fill this empty room with the joy and happiness deserving of it. My baby, my baby, my baby.

"Sweet Jesus," I prayed, "please take care of our baby, take care of our baby ... and help Helmut and me through this night."

CHAPTER FOUR

Incompatible with Nature

On the way to the clinic the following morning, my spirits were not high, but for some reason I thought everything would be okay, at least better than the dire prediction from the day before. So no, I wasn't waiting for a hammer to fall, in fact, I even thought that the results of the catheter examination would show that things weren't so bad after all. I mean, everybody can make a mistake, and perhaps the findings were not as bad as the Professor first thought. It'll be okay, I told myself. It'll be okay. It *can't* be that bad. You had the checkups.

Maybe there might be something, a little something that popped up, but it's nothing that can't be taken care of. This is your baby. He'll be fine. The German doctors with their efficiency are just doing the double-check to make sure everything's perfect. Be grateful for that. It'll be okay.

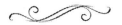

The catheterization took place later that morning. Due to the abnormalities, the procedure itself was difficult, its results nothing less than horrifying. The Professor, Helmut and I sat in a room, huddled together at a very small table.

The results of the catheterization revealed multiple, serious congenital cardiac malformations. With a single atrium and a single ventricle and pulmonary atresia, where there was no connection between the heart and the pulmonary arteries, and having no main pulmonary artery, there existed basically the absence of a normal cardiac structure; our son's tiny internal organs were simply confused. This confusion is known in the medical community as Heterotaxy syndrome. Essentially, Marc's precious heart was comprised of two chambers rather than four.

"His oxygen level is around 40-50%," the Professor said.

"So what is it supposed to be?" I asked him.

"Normally between 90-100%. There is no cure. No operation that will save the child's life," he continued. "He could live for maybe a day or two. A few weeks or a month would be highly unlikely."

I was stunned! Superior vena cava? Atrium? Ductus-dependent circulation? Small pulmonary arteries? What was he talking about? How was I supposed to deal with *this*? How on earth was I to begin to fathom what this man was telling us?

He continued talking, sometimes directing his remarks to Helmut in German. I sat forward on the edge of my chair, knees together, feet flat on the floor, hands knotted tightly in my lap. My torso rocked back and forth. A headache began to claw at my skull. God Almighty! The shock of this revelation alternately arrested and accelerated the beating of my fractured heart. I couldn't stop shivering or stop my teeth from rattling. The train had jumped the track. Everything was out of control. How could this be? He must be talking about some other baby!

It was several minutes before I could pull myself together and recover my wits enough so that I could at least be halfway coherent enough to ask him some questions, to try to make sense out of the senseless. It didn't help that I'd had little sleep, if any at all. The eventual shutting of my swollen eyelids happened long after each flower petal had quietly clenched itself together. And it hadn't been that so anticipated peaceful, placid slumber that we slip into when all is right in the world and we find ourselves floating through that unconscious land where dreams begin to brew.

No, the pitch darkness was feverish, full of fits and starts. And now deprived of my child and not knowing if I ever really got any sleep, and slowly beginning to feel like a candidate for Bedlam, I had an overwhelming urge to break out of my skin and run. Vanish! Make a beeline to the closest exit and fly like a bat out of hell away from the remnants of pregnancy, and this hospital in this foreign country with its strange language...and this matter of life and death. I'd just delivered a beautiful baby into this world; I longed to smell bouquets – instead I was being battered with bricks. I knew I would never be free again. It was now or never.

In my mind I bolted.

It didn't take long before I came to a screeching halt. Leaning forward, my hands forming a tripod with my wobbly knees, panting before a doorless entranceway, I surveyed the wide expanse of terrain before me and asked myself to which corner of the world could I run. Where would I hide? How does one run and hide from one's self?

"The truth is the light, it will set you free...don't kid yourself," Daddy's voice echoed from the recesses in my mind. The truth stung my reality; there would be no escaping. No great Houdini for me. My baby came into this world with a severe malady. This was not an illusion, no false alarm. It didn't matter that the facts were clear as mud. I didn't have a choice but to bite the bullet.

So haggard and stupid with fatigue, I asked the Professor for paper and a pen and to the best of my ability began asking questions and making notes. The terms I absolutely couldn't comprehend I asked him to write down for me. I had moved to a new world with its own language only seven months ago. I was now moving into another. From gobbledy-gook to gobbledy-gook. He put his best foot forward as far as his English was concerned.

"What causes this?" The question was presented to him simultaneously in English and German.

"We don't know," he said, and then he started speaking to Helmut in German. I cut him off.

"Does it show that he is unusually strong because he had no problems for twelve days in the hospital?"

I don't recall his answer.

"Compared with other babies with the same condition is he stronger or the same, normal or below normal?"

"There are too few children to compare him with. These babies usually die."

"Well, how long can he live with surgery?"

"Because the pulmonary artery is so small, I don't think surgery is an option for him. It will only prolong his suffering."

I had no idea what a pulmonary artery was, how big or how small it or they were supposed to be or just how important it was to the big picture. Still I tried my damnedest to keep hope alive.

"But if the pulmonary artery grew how long do you *think* he could live?" I asked him.

Avoiding my eyes, he answered with an "I don't know" shrug. I could see the lines in his forehead as his eyebrows arched for a moment under his bent head. We waited. The silence was broken by the tapping of his pen against the table. His eyes were downcast and he shook his head.

"I don't think it's possible."

Well, there had to be something damn it! I'd heard enough of all the negativism. I just couldn't believe that our son was going to *die. And soon.* And there was nothing anyone could do to prevent it? He'd just arrived! Dead is forever, beyond reckoning! There had to be *something* we could do! I needed to hear about Plan

B. This man was, after all, *the* Professor, *the* Director of Children's Cardiology at this respected hospital, *the* highest in command. He *had* to be able to show me the soothing syrup.

"So Professor, what *can* we do? Surely there must be something we can do." I had no shame begging for mercy. He could see that my heart, my spirit, that every fiber of my being bent at the knee.

"The only help is to continue the intravenous injection of the medication Prostaglandin E that we started yesterday when he was admitted to the ward. This medication is intended to keep the ductus arteriosus open."

"*Ductus?*"

"*Arteriosus.* This is an opening between the aorta and pulmonary artery which is necessary for normal fetal circulation and normally closes shortly after birth. His is still open and –"

So, if it normally closes shortly after birth and his is still open, he must be really special, I remember thinking.

"If it closes he will die," he went on. "If it stays open, then we can hope that some kind of shunting procedure may be possible. But we can't keep him on this medication too long because it causes bone and brain problems. The shunting operation would involve making an artificial communication between the aorta and the pulmonary artery. It would be difficult because the child's pulmonary artery and veins are so small. It would probably save his life, but it would not be an improvement."

"Well, if it would save his life, how could it NOT be an improvement?" I said.

"If the arteries were big enough, he could go to surgery for shunting and if that is good, he could grow to maybe six years of age. Perhaps then, a procedure called the Fontan might be carried out. But there are many complications involved. Even if he were to survive a palliative operation, which is questionable, respiratory and other infections, normal colds, fevers, as well as the risks of the surgery itself will all be problems.

"I don't see the sense in subjecting the child to pain and suffering and misery when the long-term prognosis is not good. There is no hope for him. You must understand and accept this. The best would be for us to make him as comfortable here in the hospital as possible until the time comes. He cannot thrive. He will not survive."

The Professor had transformed; he now had two heads. And for a time I left him that way, refusing to blink away the swollen rivers in my eyes. I didn't understand him. Why should I focus on him when I didn't want to see him at all, didn't want to hear another damned word of what he had to say. The tears found their familiar paths and slithered down my face.

Good grief! How were Helmut and I to deal with this? I was aware of the Professor looking straight at me, but I had again temporarily left the room, out roaming, praying, thinking, wondering, trying to understand and was not prepared for his next delivery.

"The child was born incompatible with nature," he said.

I shrunk slowly back in my chair. There was a palpable pause. His words so raw and so sharp were his final instrument of torture. *Incompatible with nature?* What did *that* mean? Was I some kind of monster? How do you look a mother in her face and utter such a thing? Where had he buried the sensitivity that should have inherently been a part of his profession, which should have accompanied the stethoscope hanging from his neck?

As a doctor, a healer, surely he could have ministered to me, this first-time mother, with no next of kin other than Helmut to support me and who himself had no one to support him, and swathed me in bandages to stem the bleeding of my heart, or massaged my scalding spirit in balm. Instead of helping me begin to scab over emotionally, he'd found the coarsest salt he had on hand and rubbed it deep in my wounds. Why didn't he just castrate me? Just start with the essence of my womanhood and tear me limb from limb until I could no longer sit in this chair and simply rose in a heap from the floor? What difference would it make?

My soul was already in tatters. And I'd been really trying. With my breasts leaking, my womb tremoring and blindly trying to find my way through this jungle, I was indeed trying. And now I hear this? Had this pit no bottom? Swallowing the bile trying to creep up my throat, my first and only thought was, *hang on, Tracie. Hang on. Only God counts the stars.*

A silent moment or two slipped by and in those few seconds I realized that he was perhaps a talented, maybe even gifted cardiologist, but he knew nothing of matters having to do with the heart. By the time all was said and done, Helmut and I were instructed to prepare for our baby's impending demise.

It was late. It helped that Marc was sleeping when we turned and walked away. I had never, ever been plunged into such profound grief. I can only describe it as an unimaginable pain outside the realms of all possibility, all reality. Up until that point, nothing in my life had been so difficult, so deeply devastating. Nothing. I thought I was dying. If there is a hell, I was surely in it. I didn't know how to handle myself in my own skin, and to make matters even worse, my psychological balance, until then always poised, teeter-tottered. I was not only a stranger in this country; I had become a stranger to myself. The cruelness about this entire scenario is that I'd had no warning, not even the slightest twinkling that this constellation coming into being within me was so critically ill. And there was no cure. It was as if there had been a confidential communication between God...and someone else.

CHAPTER FIVE

The Fight Begins

The following morning, Helmut called the hospital before daylight. There had been no changes.

I knew what lay in each cupboard, nook and cranny of our kitchen. Like every good *Hausfrau* I had taken such pride in stocking all the shelves. But I stumbled about disoriented, feeling as if I had a strong case of the flu with all the requisite muscle and joint aches, jitters and bouts of nausea.

Opening the refrigerator door, I stared inside for a moment, and then dutifully closed it. From cabinet to cabinet the same thing. Lifted the handle on the water faucet and blankly stood there watching the flow of water rush through for I don't know how long until Helmut walked in and pushed the handle down. I had planned to make him breakfast. At least my intentions were good. He ended up making it himself.

The smell of toast made me sick and sent me slowly staggering into the living room. I plopped down on the corner of the couch closest to the end table which held the telephone. It would have been unfathomable to me forty-eight hours before that on this morning my husband would be having his breakfast alone in silence, staring blankly at a butter knife rather than gazing lovingly at me and our son, and that I would be in such a state that somebody could knock me over with a feather. This bolt out of the blue so violated our euphoria it was grotesque.

He sat with me a moment before he left for work, holding me in his arms, leaning his head on mine. No words were spoken. Like a rag that's been rung, we were all talked out. He kissed my cheek as he stood to leave. His store was only a few blocks away. I remember him saying he would return in a few hours to check on me. I barely nodded my head in acknowledgement as I continued to stare blankly out the window of the sliding glass door. I sensed him pausing and turning to look at me after opening the front door. A moment later I heard a click. And with that he was gone.

I howled.

Uncorked my pain.

Let it roar from the pit of my stomach.

The shutting of the door marked the first moment that I was completely alone since this saga had begun. There was no one to observe me, no embarrassment of swollen eyes and runny nose, no stumbling over strange words, no one whose feelings I had to concern myself with but my own. I was finally free in my dungeon.

I remained fixed in my position on the couch. My legs knotted beneath me, I hugged myself and wept. Rocked back and forth, drifted wide eyed to nowhere and suddenly snapping back to the moment, began wailing and pounding my legs, whimpering, rocking, alternately feeling numb and hysterical, thinking this was somebody else's nightmare. With my breasts engorged and engulfed in a despair I had never known I breathed into each minute and wondered at the absurdity of wondering if my baby were doing the same thing: breathing.

The telephone rang half a ring.

"Maytex."

"Helmut?"

"Sweetie!"

I didn't want to call and disturb him at work and I tried to fight it, but I was losing ground and it was getting worse.

"Helmut, I...I don't think I'm gonna make it."

"Tracie, are you up? Are you dressed? Come over to me now. The couple blocks of fresh air will do you good. Come now."

To get there I only had to open the front door, go through the front gate, turn right, at the corner go right again and walk to the end of the street. There would be a stoplight in front of me and one to my left. I could either cross straight ahead with the light and walk within the confines of the crosswalk to the other side of this busy street, whereupon I would turn left at the corner and continue for three blocks straight ahead, or I could go immediately left with the other stoplight, walk the three blocks down and then cross over in the middle of the street, dodging traffic till I reached the other side.

The stoplights didn't change with the words 'walk' and 'don't walk'; traffic flowed on green, slowed on yellow, stalled on red. Just like at home. Finally reaching the corner I tried to cross on green, but I couldn't get my feet off the curb, not in one direction or the other. I knew I had two options, but I couldn't decide which way to go. So I stood there watching the lights blink traffic into command, again and again.

"Don't panic," I remember telling myself "Eventually you'll make it across. I didn't need people to think that I had also lost my mind on top of everything else. Strangers or not. Myself included. After a time, there were no cars in either direction and so I crossed straight ahead against the light on red.

When Helmut closed the store that evening, we drove directly to the hospital. There had been no change.

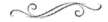

The following morning we arrived to see that Marc was no longer receiving the intravenous feeding of the Prostaglandin E though he was still connected to the heart monitor. Helmut left for work while I mothered our son the better half of the day. He looked and acted like any other baby. I dared to think about tomorrow, first steps and little bow ties. Hope gathered momentum like a steam locomotive.

The swelling began that afternoon. No one knew why. He didn't eagerly take his bottle and grew cranky. The sense of our impending loss slammed me against a wall of despair. I tried to find acceptance. If this is God's will, I thought, then so be it. It's better if it happens quickly before you really get adjusted to him, before you kiss him too much, before you dream too many dreams.

Quickly. Adjustments. Kisses. Dreams.

It wasn't working. There was no rationalizing, no pill to swallow to alleviate this nightmare or make it go away.

There were no changes throughout the night, but by the following morning, Marc looked as if he'd been pumped head to toe. He wouldn't eat. So, this is it, I remember thinking. Get ready.

I approached Heike, one of Marc's nurses. In her late twenties, of medium height and sturdy build, she was an attractive, wholesome-looking woman with a blond pixie haircut that framed her face. She had the lightest blue eyes I'd ever seen. Like they'd been infused with sunshine. The hospital staff knew I couldn't speak their language, or assumed it by looking at me, but she was one of the few I don't recall ever rushing her language past me, leaving it in a trail behind her expecting me to understand.

Her eyes locked on mine when she spoke to me. I didn't feel hurried to pick myself up when I staggered and fell trying to understand and make myself be understood. She didn't gawk at me.

I'd already found the words I wanted to say with the help of my English-German dictionary. I made her understand that I wanted Marc to be blessed by a priest. At that point, neither the denomination of the priest nor the name of the particular sacrament concerned me. The only criteria was that this person be devoutly dedicated to the service of God, and come to my son and pray for him. The clock was ticking; it had to be done immediately. I remembered Sister Mary Raymond, during one of her after-prayer oracles, declaring to my first grade class that if a baptized baby died, he wouldn't go to hell. In my mind, something would be better than nothing. Perhaps I wouldn't have the chance to protect my son in this life, but maybe I could make arrangements to guard his hereafter. And with that find myself a little peace.

My consciousness had no more space. No more room for waking nightmares. Mama always said, "God never gives us more than we can bear," and that's why I don't know who came to our son, what religion he or she represented, if he touched my baby while he prayed, what he said or how long it took to say it. I've always wondered what his face looked like. Did he smile upon my son?

Did this adult who'd been given the opportunity to reason and make choices and have a life, fill with sadness as he looked down upon my helpless baby, a child of God, my bundle of joy, all puffy and swollen? Did he know his circumstances? Could he understand that his illness could not be treated? Could he understand incompatible with nature? Were the words easier to understand in German? Did he get philosophical and pull upon the roots of his religion and think that in the end we are all born just to die anyway? Ashes to ashes?

Did he wonder where my son's mother was? If she was dead or alive? Did he wish to speak to me? Did he think he could-should-would be able to comfort me, solace me? Was he short on time? Could language have been the barrier? I'll never know.

I trusted nurse Heike to see to it that my wish would be granted, and I let it go with that. I had no choice. There comes a point when we must at some time or another be confident enough to depend upon others.

When it was over, Heike found me in the corner of a small room not far from where our son lay, standing stiff, staring out the window. The setting sun had the nerve to be a ball of gold. I didn't hear the rubber soles of her white nursing sandals when she entered the room. No words were spoken as she reached for my hand causing me to unbuckle the fists tightly bound around my waist.

Her big blue gentle eyes looked to me and then to the four-by-three inch white slip of paper she placed in my palm, then back to me. Her voice so soft I felt it more than heard it. In her native tongue she told me what she'd written on the slip of paper: "On December 18, 1984 Marc was baptized." Nurse Heike. So. It was done.

By the time Helmut arrived after work that evening, Marc's crib had been wheeled into the silence of a small empty windowless room a couple doors down from the ward. I stood at the foot of the crib and looked to the nurse locking the wheels in place.

"*Warum*?" I said, as I looked around the room, my open palms raised in wonder. Both of her hands began calmly patting at the air. I could barely hear her. "*Ruhe*," she said.

"*Ruhe*?"

"*Ruhe*. Ssh," she said.

Was she telling me to be quiet or what? A nod, a half smile that said "I'm sorry for you" and she was out the door. I grabbed my dictionary, flicking the pages until I found 'ru' then carefully traced my finger along the page until I found the word I thought she'd said. *Ruhe*: rest, repose, quiet. I then assumed that the doctors decided that his condition might improve if he could rest away from the sounds of the ward. I inhaled a deep apprehensive sigh.

Later that evening after Helmut arrived, the Professor explained to us that Marc had been placed in this room so that he would not be disturbed by the cries of the other babies when he died. When it happened, someone would call us we were promised.

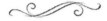

I could faintly hear the telephone ringing as Helmut unlocked the front door. A wave of heat washed over me making me dizzy. Neither of us rushed to the telephone. It had one of those rings that sounded like it would just ring itself right off the hook before the caller would replace the receiver.

"Hello? Yes, we just got home." A reprieve. I knew right away it was my family. Helmut didn't try to speak English to anybody but me or them. "No. No, there are no changes. I – we are okay. Just a minute, I give you Tracie. Yes, okay. Thank you. Bye."

"Hello?"

The voices of my parents and my two sisters thundered into their extensions all at the same time.

"Well, they think tonight will be it. He's still swollen and not eating. He was sleeping when we left. No, they still don't know why. They've moved him to a room by himself so that he . . ." I couldn't even get it out.

"Tracie, honey, now you listen to Mommy. Calm down, honey, I know."

"You don't know, Mama!"

"Tracie, if you don't calm down you're just going to make yourself sick. You are too far away for . . ."

Mama's voice blended into a chorus of words of encouragement, disbelief and confusion from my sisters.

"You'll get pregnant again," Mama said.

Sure. Just like that. And forget all this, I thought to myself.

Daddy had been strangely quiet throughout the conversation.

"Daddy, are you there?"

"I'm, uh, I'm here sugar."

"Daddy, can you help me? What do you think? How should I handle this? What should I do?"

He was quiet far too long.

Finally he said, "Baby, I'll be damned if I know what to tell you."

For the first time in my life, he didn't have the answer to the question which was the wrong answer and strangely enough, after all I'd been through, I think that was the moment I knew I was in dire straits.

He cleared his throat like he did when he was about to tell a lie or was uncomfortable.

"Perhaps you are paying for the sins of your father," he answered me.

Now, how was I to find comfort in this twisted logic? I didn't have the resources to hazard a response. He would have to deal with his own trolls and ogres; my plate was full. Anyway, whatever he meant, I didn't want to know about it. Some things are best kept to oneself.

Before I hung up, I promised to call the moment I heard something. Yes, I loved them all too.

I replaced the phone on its cradle and stared at nothing, certain that once upon a time, the world had been round.

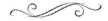

That night I took a blanket and pillow and made myself a nest in the hallway on the floor between Marc's bedroom and ours, extending the cable of the telephone from Helmut's nightstand over his body and my side of the bed so that the phone could rest on the floor by my head.

If it rang I couldn't say more than "Hello," but at least the ringing wouldn't startle Helmut awake. If someone called I could then gently rouse him. I don't know what made me think my nerves were more battle ready than his. I just knew that he had to get up and go to work and needed all of his wherewithal to function. He had to feed us.

Several hours later, I sprang up off the floor seized from a troubled slumber. That dreadful feeling of wonderful gone wrong collided with my first wakening seconds. It was not yet dawn and I knew that daylight would not bring clarity. Had I forgotten something? Where was I? How long had I been asleep? Had I slept? What time was it? Where was I? Marc! The phone! Oh my God! Could I have possibly slept through the call? Hastily fumbling with the phone I dialed the number to the hospital.

"*Kinderkardiologie Abteilung*," (Pediatric Cardiology Department) the voice said.

"Hello? This is Tracie Mayer. I call for my son Marc."

I didn't understand her response, but instinctively I felt that if something terrible had happened, she was talking too long about it. And her voice was lilting.

"Wait!" I screamed into the phone. "Please wait!"

Helmut snapped awake, propped himself up on his elbow and faced me. Leaping onto the bed and cradling the receiver at his ear, my voice trembling so I could barely speak, I said, "What's she saying, Helmut? What's she saying?"

He sat up straight in the bed and tried to shush me with his hands. As he spoke into the phone he stopped midway into the formalities. The nurse obviously let him know she knew with whom she was speaking. Slowly he began to smile. That's all I needed.

"I knew it! I knew it!" I started screaming over and over again as I snatched my jogging suit out of the closet cabinet and pulled it on over my pajamas.

"Marc! Hang on, honey! Mommy's on her way! Hang on!" I dove down the fourteen stairs to the living room three, four at a time. I was out the front door and on the way to our baby before Helmut had even hung up the phone.

My fight for our son's life had begun.

CHAPTER SIX

Heirlooms

A two-time beauty queen, one of Mama's coronations distinguishes her as the first black beauty queen in her hometown of Seattle, Washington. Daddy blew into her emerald city from Detroit, Michigan. Mile-long canary yellow convertible Cadillac and all.

A continuous hubbub of excitement permeated the air of the auditorium on that balmy summer evening in 1950. Anxiously waiting in the wings, Mama directed her gaze towards the trio assembled rear center stage. She watched Daddy bob his head to a count of three whereupon his teardrop-tipped drumsticks made a sound, the right sound, giving his bandmates their cue.

Before the evening had come to an end, forty five contestants had strutted back and forth across the stage to various thunders of applause. As the Master of Ceremonies prepared to call out the name of the winner, Daddy's sticks rolled across the drums heightening the anticipation. Mama could walk her talk. And she did as she glided triumphantly in strappy high heels and a white one-piece bathing suit across the stage to pick up her second beauty title, Miss Bronze of Seattle. Her lips, the same intense hue as the hibiscus pinned above her breast, looked as though they'd be red forever. Aside from his mother, she was the most divine woman Daddy had ever seen. He dropped anchor.

This dynamo intimidated but intrigued Mama, a self-sure, but sheltered young woman. After playing a little hard to get, she finally consented to a date and with that their courtship began.

It was short lived. Daddy got drafted. During his stint in the army, he won the first Civil Rights lawsuit in the state of Washington to go to Superior Court. The fact that he and his fellow black soldiers could be sent off to war, yet be denied the freedom to sit at public lunch counters in the city of their posting base in Tacoma, Washington was intolerable.

Mama said that he could charm a bird out of a tree. They married in February 1956. When I arrived the following year, Mama said that Daddy was thrilled. A girl! But I do believe that I was supposed to have been a boy! The one my father always wanted. It was a family joke that hinted towards the truth: my father wanted his eldest child to be a male.

When I emerged from my mother's womb with a vagina instead of a penis, she says he poked his chest out and wore a Cheshire cat grin. I'm inclined to think that if he could have chosen my sex chromosome, he would have bestowed upon his woman a 'man child' and thereby ensured the succession of the family heirlooms. After the birth of my second and youngest sister, he would look at his three offspring and shake his head in mock defeat. Mama couldn't resist the opportunity to instigate. "It takes a man to make a boy, Gerald," she'd say.

Daddy was the powers that be. Though he loved my sisters, Mama and me dearly, he did not hesitate to remind us that we had to "stay in our place" (wherever that was, it was not a space occupied by men), that he was the only one in our house "who could think" and that we'd better never assume we could "outthink" him, and we'd "better pick up a book and read goddamnit!" His cramped ideas about womankind in general determined us inadequate, inferior. Mentally dull.

He opined that women as a species suffered from "bitchology". My mother included. Occasionally he plucked my sisters and me out of this group; instances when he believed that our ability to function didn't stem from a knee-jerk response. After all, we came from "good stock" and he expected nothing less. I remember those times when he was proud of something I'd done, how he would wrap his arm around my shoulder and hammer the thumb of his free hand back and forth against his chest and boast, "That's my child! I didn't raise no dummies!" How I beamed!

Being the oldest had its advantages and disadvantages. My father's monumental expectations compelled me to jump through high loops. Sometimes laced in fire. As my successes mounted, my freedom and independence were encouraged. Mama said the world was at my fingertips. Daddy said it was just that way shy of the stars. Reach!

Though I always tried to be the best child and young adult that I could be, I always felt that in his eyes, I came up short. Ninety-nine was good – but it was no cigar. Perhaps this was his way of trying to pull the best out of me, to make me challenge myself to the nth degree, to be as brave and strong and knowing as I at one time thought him to be. Did he foresee something? Even if he dared to suspect the day would come that a will of my own would eventually steer my vision beyond his horizons, he certainly couldn't have imagined the road that lay before me.

While he prepared his daughter to live in what he referred to as a man's world, my mother instilled a certain womanliness in me. Though she grew up in a house with too few bedrooms for too many children, she carried herself with a noble bearing. A natural, confident sense of style told you she knew where she was going, even if she didn't. Never afraid to get down in the trenches, yet she always took the time to ensure her perfume suited the seasons, instinctively knowing that less is more. The aroma of whatever she had simmering on the stove greeted you at the front door, made you happy to be home. She was what I like to call a woman's woman.

Daddy used to give her behind an affectionate pat and call her Prissy Missy, the only way he knew how to tell her that he admired her gumption as well as her long manicured fingernails. And though he liked to play "Me Tarzan, You Jane", deep in his heart he knew that Mama was a fierce protector and the bedrock of our family.

As a child, she symbolized everything that was right in my world. Her belief in her faith never wavered; "Let go and let God" she'd say. Come hell or high water she affirmed the hopeful; her positive way of thinking was shatterproof. Always in my corner, ninety-nine wasn't just the cigar, it was the whole damn tobacco harvest. She was for me that comforting cup of cocoa you sip, then close your eyes, wiggle your toes and say "yum." Whereas Daddy's scalded, causing you to jerk your head back from the cup and say "damn!" Though I knew the burn wouldn't subside for days, I continued slurping air with peanut-sized mouthfuls of steaming liquid, unable to set my cup down. Somehow he just motivated, if not dared me to be up to the challenge. His "if you ain't got no heart, you might as well be dead" attitude, high intellect, and outrageous banter drew people to him like a magnet. He was the full three hundred and sixty degrees. As a child I thought he could make cows fly. It seems all my life I strove to meet his expectations.

Until he succumbed to alcohol and manic-depression which created a permanent intermission between he and myself, and ultimately destroyed the family. Fortunately, before Daddy's shipwreck, my parents had instilled within me the mental munitions that would help sustain me those days and nights I fought to hold on in a whirlwind of pain and confusion.

I had indeed inherited the family heirlooms. Powder keg and all.

CHAPTER SEVEN

Destiny

I was born and raised in that Pacific Northwest region of America where my parents first met. Affectionately known to its inhabitants as the Emerald City, Seattle is surrounded by nearly 200 miles of water and the Washington Cascades, part of the Cascade Mountain Range which extends from British Columbia to California. A good deal of the city's attraction lies in the stunning views from various neighborhood vantage points.

The house I called home the last nineteen years I lived in America was located in a dead end. Literally. It was the only house on 33rd and Yesler, a street which ran all the way downtown to 1st and Yesler, the historic part of the city called Pioneer Square. Our home towered over a cliff, and nearly every room had its own breathtaking view of Lake Washington, the old floating bridge, rows of mountain ranges as well as that majestic volcano Mount Rainier.

For twelve years, from Monday through Friday, except for the occasional free dress day, I wore black or saddle oxford shoes, white or navy blue knee-high socks (in high school, navy or black stockings), a plaid blue and gray pleated skirt, a white blouse and blue cardigan to school. Upon graduating from high school with a B average, I attended Seattle University and received a degree in Business Administration. My greatest desire to study journalism was a red flag to a bull in Daddy's eyes and he was paying my tuition fees so that took care of that issue.

The two rental properties my father owned when he married my mother would eventually over a span of twenty-five years snowball into nearly four hundred. Everybody had to earn their keep. I entered at the grass roots level, literally.

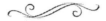

"Well, good afternoon."

I peeled open an eye and looked at the clock on my nightstand. It was seven in the morning. Saturday morning. I closed my eye.

"Mornin' Daddy. What do you want?"

"Sugar, I need you to get up and get dressed. I'm'll have to drop you off at the apartments over on 16th. We've got to pull some weeds and pick up the cigarette butts and empty bottles in the yard. Get the place spruced up a bit."

"Okay, but let me sleep one more hour," I said snuggling further down into the warmth of my bed.

"One more hour? The day's already almost over. You got to get up and get on it. Come on now. Get up and get your clothes on. I'll be waiting for you in the kitchen. You want some breakfast?"

"Uh-uh, no thanks." I lay there a couple more minutes curled tight, hugging my sheet, blanket and bedspread around my neck, savoring those last minutes of cozy. I knew I'd have to get up sooner rather than later. Might as well just get it over with. Reluctantly I threw the covers off and wiped the sleep from my nine-year-old eyes. Got to get up and get on it.

Within the half hour Daddy had rolled our blue Volkswagen bus to a stop in front of the four-unit building. I hopped out armed with a roll of extra-strength blue plastic sacks, a rake, a broom and dustpan, a pair of rubber gloves, and his instructions.

"Now you just walk around the building and you'll see the stuff that has to be picked up. Try to get as close to the roots of the weeds as you can. I'll be back to check on you in a couple of hours."

I settled my tools against the front stairs and looked around the yard. I didn't know where to start but I knew I'd better start somewhere because Daddy would be back soon to check and I wanted him to think I'd done a good job.

I ripped a sack away from the roll and dragged it alongside me as I waded through the uneven growth. I hated it, but hating it was not going to pick up all the garbage. With the tips of my gloved fingers I picked up the cigarette butts, dirty tissues and empty cans and bottles and tossed them inside. Holding my breath I scraped dog poop with the tines of the rake onto the dustpan and dropped it in the bag. I had to get all that out of the way before I could start pulling weeds.

Over the years, I progressed from cleaning the yards and parking lots to filthy ovens and refrigerators. I quickly learned to scour dirty sinks and ring-rimmed bathtubs until they would look as though they'd been licked. There was no point in doing a less than perfect job because I would have to stay until whatever I was cleaning was clean. And that would mean staying all day if necessary. By the time I graduated from college I worked in the office full time.

By 1982, Frank Enterprises was at its zenith. Life began and ended with the business. Period. Over the years Daddy added on extensions to the main house, so that eventually my two sisters and I each had our own apartment overlooking the pool as well as direct access to the office which protruded from the front of the house. No reason for me to be in there a minute later than 7:31 in the morning, waiting for the crew with their detailed job descriptions for the day. And they'd "better" be in their designated trucks with addresses, keys and maintenance materials and gone up the hill by 8:15 A.M. because "by 8:20 the day is half over!"

"Frank Enterprises, good morning."

"Yes, I'm calling about your ad for the apartment on Capitol Hill."

"Fine. I'll meet you outside the building at two o'clock."

"Frank Enterprises."

"Is this here Frank Enterprises?"

"Yes, Mrs. Anderson, this is Tracie."

"Tracie?"

"Yes, Mrs. Anderson, what can I do for you?"

"Well, honey, I just want to tell you that those kids were runnin' up and down these halls ALL night long again last night and honey you know I need my rest and I just don't understand it."

"Mrs. Anderson—"

"And honey you know I pay my rent just like everyb—"

"Mrs. Anderson, I promise I'll speak with their mother again. Thanks for calling."

"Yeah?"

"This is Tracie Frank calling. Anthony is that you?"

Silence.

"Anthony look – I am busy. Now answer me! Is that you?"

"Yeah."

"Were you kids running up and down the halls again last night?"

"I don't know."

"Let me speak with your mother."

"She's not here."

"When will she be back?"

"I don't know."

"Where is she?"

"I don't know."

"Frank Enterprises."

"This is Ruth from your Seattle City Light calling. You had a tenant move out sometime last month. We're trying to locate this person. Would you please check your records for his forwarding address – I'll hold."

"Ruth, this will be a minute. I've got a call on the other line."

"Mr. Smith, this is Tracie Frank calling again about your delinquent rent. You don't have it isn't good enough, Mr. Smith. I'll have the carpenter pick you up on his way into the office tomorrow morning and we'll make arrangements for you to begin working off your rent. No, Mr. Smith, I do not want to hold your television until you get the money together. I'll see you at seven forty-five in the morning."

"Ms. Frank, we need an okay to make a copy of these keys..."

"Tracie, we ran out of the oyster white flat paint, Are you sure we're supposed to knock down that wall between the bedroom and the closet?"

"Yes Daddy, the evictions are ready. I'll be in court at eleven-thirty day after tomorrow."

"Okay, that's fine, sugar. Now this afternoon while you're out, stop by 17th and tell that crazy woman in number 302 that her boyfriend is subletting. His name is not on the lease so either she's gonna have to pay more rent or he's got to go. And I want his raggedy-ass car out of the parking lot today. I made an appointment for you to show number 306 at four-fifteen this afternoon so you can do it then. And before you come in, swing by Spring Street and see how the fellas made out. I want them to get finished with the detailing of that unit so it can be rented before the end of the week. Oh! Did you get that letter off to the people down on the Lake property notifying them of their rent increase? And don't forget now, after the crew gets outta here in the morning I'm gonna need you to go down to the Millionaire's Club and pick up a couple extra laborers for some yard detail..."

"Mr. McAdams, as director of this bank, located in the heart of the central area of our beautiful city, I implore you to reconsider your 'unofficial' practice of redlining in this area and release the requested funds for the upgrading of the aforementioned property. Our community desperately needs and has the right to clean and affordable housing."

"This letter says that McAdams has again denied our application, Daddy."

"That stupid jackass. Okay, sugar. We'll have picket signs outside the bank tomorrow morning. First thing. And tomorrow evening we'll carry them in front of his lily white house in his lily white neighborhood. You have the best penmanship. I want "Unfair! Beware!" printed in big bold red and black letters. We'll get the refinancing. You just listen to your daddy . . ."

All typical do-this-do-that occupy yourself with a person, place and thing days. Oftentimes, it seemed there weren't enough hours between sunrise and sunset, and by the end of the day I felt like I'd been spread like butter. When I finally silenced the office with a flick of the light switch, daddy would flick it back on, ready for a gabfest, whiskey and coke in hand.

"Daddy, I've had enough for one day."

Ignoring me, he would take a seat in the swivel chair behind the desk and prepare to hold court.

"I've got some information here for you, so you better sit down and listen to me. The business must go on. Ain't no givin' up and no givin' out. Now listen . . ."

"Daddy, I can't hear it anymore! Enough for one day is enough! If you want blood you're gonna have go to the Red Cross!"

"Stay stupid, then you damn dummy!"

I sat.

By the end of December 1982, the demands of the business and never knowing if my father's spirit would be in the sky or in the sewer had me fatigued. It didn't take much convincing for a high school girlfriend to talk me into a first of the year three-day jaunt to Puerto Vallarta, Mexico. Just to relax and spend a few perfect days under the sun. Now, under no circumstances would three days be stretched into four. I'd have to be back by the third of January. Rents were due on the first. Late-fee notices went out on the fifth.

As the plane touched down in Mexico, I had no idea that the itinerary of my life was about to change. Destiny happens when we least expect it. She has a magnetic force, she is inescapable.

CHAPTER EIGHT

A Flicker of Promise

Just as mysteriously as Marc's swelling started, it stopped. As I raced onto the first floor of the hospital, one of the station nurses smiled and pointed me in the direction of the ward. There he was taking his bottle in the arms of a nurse. I threw on the mandatory green dressing gown and took over the feeding. I was thrilled down to my very bones.

Helmut came up sometime later that morning. He just couldn't believe it. Our son looked like our son again. I was convinced that this was a direct sign from God and an indication of our son's fighting spirit. We met the Professor in his office. He didn't agree with me.

"I don't know what the swelling meant or why it is gone," he said. "But it doesn't change anything."

"But he's eating and acting normal again," I said.

"It won't last," he said. "It's not possible."

His eyes didn't hold even the tiniest flicker of promise. Moored so firmly to his position, he sucked the wind right out of my sails. To all my intents and purposes, dragging out this conversation would be a wasted effort. He clearly was not inclined towards saying anything I wanted to hear. And likewise, he knew that I didn't want to hear anything he had to say. The battle line had been drawn. And each breath Marc took deepened it and lengthened it and made it wider. I clung to the fact that as long as my baby was alive I would be on a mission. I could not afford to sit on the sidelines and I would not. As far as I was concerned, the Professor needed to get some team spirit.

Pinching the bridge of my nose, trying somewhat successfully to stop myself from crying, I quietly stood, excused myself from his office and headed back to Marc.

Deflated but not defeated. I had hope because my son was alive.

What else was there?

Helmut had gone back to work. I leaned back into the hardness of the chair placed next to Marc's bed and rested my hand on top of the crib coverlet somewhere near his feet as he slept. My gaze drifted beyond the windowpanes to that point where the horizon melted into the sky...

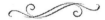

Bare feet. Warm sand. Palm-fringed beaches. Puerto Vallarta.

Though the beachfront restaurant was comfortably crowded, my girlfriend Valerie and I spotted a free table not far from the water's edge and moseyed on over. I didn't have a care in the world while we waited on our orders, laughing and rehashing all the events of the past two days when suddenly I looked up directly into Helmut's face. Did a double take. He likes to say that I winked at him. I could swear it was just the sun in my eyes.

He was in a cluster of guys, each of whom had sprawled himself picture-postcard perfect in the sand or in one of the low-backed sun chairs belonging to the adjacent beachside bar. While the guys tried to get our attention, Valerie and I chatted away. But he and I were alone at the beach; we made eyes with each other. Penetrating glances where time stopped. Again and again. Something was going to happen. I knew it.

He headed towards me. I scooted up and sat perched on the edge of my chair, smiling in his direction, my arms folded across each other on the table. Aside from the blue in his midnight blue bikini swim trunks, he was golden, from head to foot. With the last step of his approach he eased himself into bent knee alongside me. He crouched so close we could've touched toes if we dared.

In halting English he said, "Hi. My name is Helmut."

"Hi, I'm Tracie. Where are you from?"

"I am from Germany, and you?"

"My girlfriend and I are from Seattle, Washington. We're on the northwest coast of America, neighbors with Canada," I said, positioning my hands in the air on an invisible map indicating the positions of the states along the west coast of America. He stayed about ten minutes and we made that sort of conversation people make when they first meet each other. And want to see each other again. Only we spoke slower and used our limbs a lot. His buddies began ribbing him from across the way. They didn't believe he'd have the nerve to come over to our table. He chuckled and threw a glance their way over his shoulder. He looked back to me and our giggles were tinged a soft shade of crimson in the sunlight.

"Tonight you meet me?" he said. His eyes shimmered gold and green and brown.

"Well, we're invited to a party and –"

"Before the party we meet at Carlos O'Brian's disco. Eight o'clock?" he said.

"Okay, I'll meet you there." I said.

He reluctantly stood to leave and our eyes feverishly held fast.

That night he spotted Valerie and me on the ragged edges of the forefront of the line outside the disco that had no end in sight. He maneuvered his way between the throng of people and pulled us inside. We made our way to his table, one of what seemed like hundreds stretching from here to there packed with party people. His arm enveloped my waist before we sat down. The club photographer captured our kilowatt smiles. Somehow, we settled into our own little pocket of conversation. We would meet later that evening at another club.

The wee hours of the morning saw him pull me tight into his arms in the middle of the dance floor. "Now you stay with me," he said.

And we danced and danced and by the time the sun had risen...

"Frau Mayer...Frau May—"

I snapped my head to attention.

"Es ist Zeit," ("It's time"), the nurse said handing me the thermometer. Embarrassed, yet somewhat annoyed that I'd been disturbed, I nonetheless smiled up at her.

"Thank you," I said, hoping that I didn't look a fool lost in my private dream in this public place. Time to take Marc's temperature. I laid the thermometer on a towel near where he lay. I would wait just a little longer; he would soon stir.

CHAPTER NINE

Defiance

I'm extremely happy I did not become suicidal. I heard no carols, threw no streamers at midnight, blew out no candles, and ate no cake. The sterile walls of the University clinic eclipsed all celebratory events. Bliss had been replaced by brouhaha.

Alone, afraid and even though we'd been in the hospital for nearly a month, my maternal instincts continued to shilly-shally, unsure if they were in or out of a job as the just being there tested all the confidence I had as to whether or not I was tilting the bottle just right and if I was certain that burp was loud enough or if the poops were the right color and all the while I was constantly vexed by a host of questions, the main one unrelenting in its throbbing against the membranes of my skull: Is everything okay or is something wrong? I was in a state of constant alert.

Though it was my only salvation, my breathing became labored just from the thought of flipping through the pages of my pocket dictionary. Those first weeks I only did so when dire need left me no choice because by the time I'd find all the words of my sentence fragment and fragment is what it would be, making my illiterate-sounding self seem coherent to a doctor or nurse who made me feel like I'd better hurry up and spit out whatever it was I was trying to say, was simply too taxing. It was imperative that I keep an even keel at all costs so it was just less tug on my sensibilities to figure things out myself. I also discovered this to be a very good way to stay focused and not have time to wallow in what could not help me.

The residue of continuing to manage with so many foreign elements in a catatonic state led me to develop an irritating quirk. Or shall I say succumb to it. Double-checking; sort of a defense mechanism whereby I sought the certainty in, of and about everything. If I was sure of it, I could put it away and move on to the next high jump.

Easierly. But my efforts were often thwarted and not by some outside force. The problem was that my thought processes galloped like wild horses on the wind. Trying to get on top of a myriad of things fueled the impetus of my mental activity to the point that by the time I'd finally sputter out a question, I'd already have hit a blank wall. I couldn't grasp a complete understanding of the answer because I was trying to comprehend its formulating words as well as trying to remember how the words were put together and in the same moment familiarize myself to their guttural yet at times melodious sound as well as decipher deadpan facial expressions in addition to seeking clues from the pointing of fingers here and there, having prefixed all this beforehand of course with the decision to make the most of the moment while I had someone's attention and find the starting point in my mind to the next question, just forget about all the other zillion little fidgeters flitting about in my head.

Basically, I was a goner. So when I didn't hear the person speaking anymore, I'd find myself saying, *"Bitte?"*; in other words, "I beg your pardon?" In my mind, I was trying to assemble the whole shebang and stay focused on just the answer. To get around the fidgeters it was better to double-check and make sure I understood what was being said to me, and even if I didn't understand all the words comprising the answer, if the answer felt right or seemed logical, then it was a safe bet that my question had been correctly understood and I could file the whole thing away. I think the high stakes quickened my insight.

I didn't have time for a course in German so I had to learn by osmosis. Quite honestly, this double-checking is nothing that I wouldn't do in my own language, especially if it pertained to a serious matter. I mean, if I err, please let it not be on the side of negligence. More often than I care to recall, to my request of *"Bitte?"*, I got the following reply: *"Ich habe es Ihnen doch gerade erklärt."* ("I just explained it to you.") To add insult to injury he or she would then stare at me incredulously. The last time somebody stated this to me I said, "Tracie, honey, unh-uh. You don't need this extra anxiety from these exalted blockheads. Why bother?"

Some things, like the traits of poops, reveal themselves over the course of a short amount of time.

Just have to pay attention to any irregularities. No pun intended.

Their behavior was a clear manifestation of restraint; as though they had been warned: don't wet-nurse or encourage her, keep your distance, she's taboo. I don't know, looking back, perhaps I took it too personally, but I doubt it. I distinctly remember feeling being treated like a pariah from the majority of the staff. I couldn't figure out how to look in their lamentable eyes. I didn't like what I saw there before they quickly blinked away.

Everyone seemed so stoic, as if bereft of their senses, emotionally anesthetized. What was wrong with these people? I recognized that Marc and I weren't the only patients in the ward and I didn't expect anybody to hold my hand or do me any favors, but goodness gracious, a bit of compassion would have done wonders for my confidence and ability to cope.

It didn't take long before I realized that my reasonable expectation of empathy would not be forthcoming and I wondered how I would feel in a hospital in my own country. I'm convinced that even if I were deaf and mute I could not have possibly felt so isolated. The only one I could lean on was Helmut and he wasn't there all day, so that left me with...me.

The only place to go was inside. On tiptoe. This was after all very shaky ground, replete with booby traps, land mines and cliffs; thoroughly unfamiliar territory. The tactician in me detailed my blueprint.

"Okay. Now look. Let's just take this one step at a time, Tracie," I told myself. "That's it, take it easy, take it easy. Breathe. We're gonna do this real slow, even if we have to do it minute by minute."

"Listen. You cannot change this situation, neither can you believe this has happened, but it has and now you and you alone must deal with it. You're gonna have to get a grip."

"How am I supposed to deal with something I don't understand?"

"First of all, Daddy didn't 'raise no dummies'. Secondly, who do you think you are that you have to understand everything? And even if you could understand the extraordinariness of this event, what difference would it make? What would it change? Marc would still be your baby, he would still be ill, your dreams would still be scattered like leaves, you would still be in this country, you would still not know a soul, you still wouldn't be able to speak the language, you'd still feel like you appear as if you'd swallowed a stupid pill when someone speaks to you, Helmut would still have to work all day and you would STILL be alone to deal with this by yourself. You'll deal with it because you have no other options. This was your choice. You wanted to come to Germany."

"My God, what was I thinking?"

"What were you thinking? You weren't! You fell in love. Couldn't wait to have a baby. Now you've got your love, you've got your baby. This is your world so welcome to it. Things aren't going as you planned, but sometimes the best-laid plans go awry and life isn't going to allure you or anybody else with one come hither look after another and there will be days the sun won't shine goddamn it! But what are you gonna do?

"There are cloudbursts and cloudscapes and both will take your breath away. And no matter how sorry you're feeling for yourself, you'd better believe that nobody, but nobody makes it from A to Z in this life in a vapor of frankincense and myrrh. Sometimes we have to damn near squeeze our noses so tight they just about pop off our faces because life reeks like stinking rotten eggs. You don't need a mystic vision to see that.

"So pull yourself together and do it now. It's a new day and you got up, got cracking, outfitted yourself with an 'I believe smile' on your face, marched up the flight of stairs to this ward and without respite you engage yourself with the business of tending to your son like you've been doing every day for weeks now. Don't stop shaking your fist at them! The nonbelievers. The naysayers. The he-will-die sayers.

"It may not be apparent to you, but your mettlesome spirit and Marc's stamina, his declaration, no, his demand that he be contended with, mince no words. It is with one voice that you and your child tell them to stick their pessimism right up there where the sun doesn't shine. Such effrontery! You know the white coats don't like that. But they don't know that you come from a long line of warriors: 'Ain't no givin' up and no givin' out.'

"Under absolutely no circumstances will you give up on your child and live out the rest of your days stooping through life, having nothing to say for yourself. It's not even a consideration. You don't need anybody's sympathy. Let these doctors keep their gloomy bullshit on their side of the fence. You've got all the support you need, well, maybe not all you need, but it's certainly all you're gonna get around here so get yourself together. Flexibility is a major component of war and you, my friend, are in battle. You're on a mission of a lifetime."

I did my best to find comfort within myself and with prayer. "Dear God," I prayed. "This is a matter of life and death and as long as my baby is alive I will allow nothing nor no one to destroy me. He needs me. Lord, help me. Give me the wherewithal to be up to this challenge. Empower me to be resilient in this maelstrom. Command my inner resources to fortify me on all fronts, make me strong, make me strong, make me strong and if I can't move this mountain of adversity, Lord, then please, just please help me to climb it."

Whew. Some days I thought I'd go mad and had to keep reminding myself that the nonstop waves of confusion and fear did not constitute a disorder. Eventually I came to believe and accept that they comprised part of the package. Indeed, they were quite suitable for the situation and I realized that if at times I didn't think I was losing my mind, then I was really psychotic. I remember Dr. Gillor suggesting to me that I seek psychological counseling.

"Do you know anyone who could help me in English?" I asked him.

"No," he said.

So that meant that I would have to go through the drudgery of choosing a therapist who could best serve my needs, which meant of course I'd have to first decipher the Ph.D.'s from the M.D.'s from the Psy.D.'s and so on; distinguish the difference between registered and licensed and decide which certificate denoted a better therapist and just not to waste anybody's time, immediately ask and consider how well he or she answered my first question: "What expertise do you have with my type of problem?"

Wading through the psychoanalysis process in German didn't even come into question. My body was experiencing hormonal shifts readjusting itself back to my pre-pregnancy state but this tumult had nothing to do with postpartum depression. I had to get myself together. Plain and simple. Yesterday.

"Okay Tracie," I said. "You know you're distressed and you know the cause of your distress. If you're leaving any footprints on the ceiling, you have a right to, damn it. You don't have to apologize or make excuses to anybody for anything. The only way to restore your emotional well-being is to immerse yourself completely in Marc's survival. The only way. This is not a multiple choice. So stop your bellyaching and get on with it. Sniveling will not, I repeat, will not change anything."

Facing down the albatross was all I could do. Uncertainty kept my heart aflutter and sometimes I would catch myself saying, "Inhale. Exhale. Now swallow." But I began to arrive at the hospital each morning, my eyes a little less swollen than the day before, anxiously looking forward to the joys of motherhood. I decided that I would be the channel through which Marc would perceive calm and contentment. Through me he would know that all was right with the world. Under no circumstance should he sense an inkling of the absolute raw terror piercing the nerves beneath my skin.

The staff must have thought me insane in my green robe, rendering poetic license to the tending of my baby, uninhibitedly swaddling him in maternal affection. Numerous days, with a hand towel on my shoulder, I'd cup his head with my hand and nestle him to my neck. We'd gently bounce and swing from side to side as far away from the heart monitor machine as its leash would allow and back, for hours, me continuously whispering that affectionate sugar coated talk only mothers talk, and sometimes, depending on his response, finding myself getting quite animated.

While feeding and diapering, I sang songs to him, asked him questions, told him about me, his papa, his family in America. I told him when the sun was shining and that my love for him was even bigger than that fiery red circle around it. I told him about the rain and how it made my hair frizzy but was good for the ducks. I prayed with him. In our little corner of the ward I tried to provide a climate of emotional warmth for him. And me. All the while nurturing him under curious eyes pretending not to watch.

That's what I hated the most, even more than the actual being there: each hurdle I leaped at the onset of motherhood was observed by others. There was no opportunity for privacy.

But soon, even that was okay because I had a secret.

Day after day, my son displayed an instinct for pulling out the mother in me. His strength made my courage incontestable, my resolve more determined. There was no way on this planet I would let him down. In my mind, every gurgle and every smile was a magic carpet ride closer towards home. So as rough as things were, I couldn't help but be encouraged when darkness would begin to set upon our evenings. It was usually around midnight when I kissed him goodnight. There were only a few hours until morning. Let them get an eyeful.

Though he wasn't getting the medication to keep his ductus open, it didn't close. And didn't close and didn't close and Marc didn't die. And didn't die and didn't die. This ran absolutely contrary to what the doctors kept telling me. Before I knew it, weeks rolled into more weeks. I was so thankful to have a routine I didn't even realize how quickly it had established itself. Struggling against the circumstances, I just kept telling myself, "It ain't no givin' up and no givin' out."

Marc defied the doctors while my days defied the imagination.

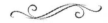

I literally shot out of bed every morning around six. Thrilled because there were no distressing phone calls during the night, I found myself in traffic no later than 6:40.

I remember, one crisp gray morning when I still didn't quite have my locality bearings, deciding to take a shortcut. Though I didn't notice it at the time, I ended up on a street with a narrow blue and white traffic sign that read *Einbahnstrasse*. Even if I would have noticed it, I wouldn't have understood what it said anyway. Without warning, a great big thick shiny beige-colored Mercedes taxi came barreling down the street seemingly out of nowhere, directly headed towards the nose of my car.

"So what's wrong with this guy? Is he stupid or what?" I remember thinking. I slowed and steered my car to the right side of the road. He stretched his arm out the window and began frantically pointing at the street, his contorted face jabbering. Did he know I was lost? Unlikely. Was he trying to help me get to the hospital? Even more so. Just what I needed: a nutcase before noon.

I didn't know what he wanted – but whatever it was I didn't have time for it. I put the pedal to the metal and drove on. Aside from the supersonic speed allowed for on the Autobahn, the rules of traffic here vary only slightly from those stateside and at the time interested me about as much as dirt under a stranger's fingernail, so I didn't think anymore about the incident. I didn't take that 'shortcut' again. It turned out to be way too long. A fine cold sweat trickled down my back by the time I finally found the hospital.

Many months later, I found myself again on this same street. I laughed out loud at the memory of the taxi driver. Jabber, jabber, jabber! Probable translation:

"Lady are you crazy? Can't you see you're driving the wrong way on a one-way street?"

It would be usually just around seven when I would be forced to slow to a stop in front of a long red and white parking lot barrier gate at the south-side parking entrance of the hospital grounds. When I rolled down my window to address the guard, that warm, delectable aroma of freshly baked *Brötchen* and strong hot coffee emanating from the little kiosk nearby greeted me with open arms. Just the sight of him irritated me. It wasn't necessary to come shuffling towards me; we could duel from his perched position in the little guardhouse.

Between drags on his Marlboros, the most important moments of his day must have revolved around those times he decided for whom he would push his little button, thereby raising the barrier gate to allow visitors to park on the grounds of the hospital. Or for whom he would not. If the bar wasn't raised, the results guaranteed a time-consuming search for a parking spot that could end up being anywhere upwards of two blocks away from the grounds of the clinic. Now, I tried to give him the benefit of the doubt. I even tried to assume that he was important to this whole hospital scenario. I wanted to give him some respect because every job should be respected, but after weeks of this nonsense I'd had enough.

"*Guten Morgen,*" he said, resting his arm on the roof and leaning into my half-opened window.

"*Guten Morgen,*" I said, looking straight ahead. "Mayer. My son. *Kinderkardiologie.* Professor." A nod of my head and an index finger lifted in the direction of my intent was meant to confirm that we'd done this before; I knew where I was going and where to park so he should just hurry up and lift the bar.

"There are only a few parking places this morning," he said. This is what he always said those mornings he'd fallen out the wrong side of the bed.

I'd already explained several times already that my child was laying in the *Kinderkardiologie* department under the care of the Professor. This buffoon knew me. It thoroughly angered me that he wielded this authority over me. Based solely on his mood. On his good days, he'd stay seated in his box, not even lift his head my way and the bar would raise before I'd even come to a full stop in front of it. It was seven in the morning. I knew there were parking places. He knew I knew he knew there were parking places. Enough. There always were.

"Let me in," I told him. "If I park wrong then tow my car away, but I must get to my baby." I lost five pounds just trying to get that out coherently and succinctly.

He stared at me for a moment. This was beyond frustrating. Why did I have to deal with this dullard? Didn't I have enough? I stared at the bar. Finally it began to rattle upwards. Before it had fully raised, I roared through, my tires screeching as I slammed on the brakes careening the car to the left before coming to an abrupt stop that propelled me and the car quickly to and fro.

As usual I parked in that area behind the building where my son lay. And as usual, at this time of the morning, I easily found a parking place. The frustration of not being able to verbalize myself swiftly and accurately was beginning to put a great big evil chip on my shoulder. This kind of irritation was not conducive to me starting off my day on a good note which in turn was not good for Marc which of course meant it had to be eliminated. So many times after Marc had fallen asleep I found myself sitting next to his crib with my dictionary in hand, imagining different scenarios and jotting down snatches of what I would say the next time I had to confront this idiot.

But not anymore. I hope he enjoyed it because today was it. This was the last time this ignoramus would wave his "I'm important" banner atop my head. I hadn't complained up until now because they all had me thinking that each day here would be my last. Well. It looked to me like I was going to be here for a while so I sought out the Professor.

"Professor, every morning I have a problem being able to park here behind the building. Is there a document or a parking sticker available for me so that I can freely park here on the hospital grounds in the morning without having to talk to the guard about it?"

I didn't even bother going into the details. I could have surely told him that the guy was a moron who decided at whim for whom he would lift the bar and what a goddamn headache it was for me each and every morning to have to explain myself and why I was here and where I was going. Priorities took on a new meaning in my life. As much as I wanted to get this man fired, I realized that that would not necessarily help my situation. What I needed was a signature of authority on a piece of paper that I could put in the front window of my car saying "Let her park here. With no hassle." Just a little 3x3 inch piece of white paper could give me peace.

"Visitor" it said in red blocked letters. Underneath, the Professor's scribbly scrawly signature.

Though revenge is not a good thing, it can be sweet.

The next morning I didn't even give him the courtesy of rolling down my window. I eased right up to the gate until my headlights were not even inches away from it. Weary Willy stood up in his little Cracker Jack box booth and languorously approached my window as if he deliberately refused to be hurried. Mr. Important. About to lose his pants and he didn't even know it.

Our eyes locked for but a moment. Um-hmm. I pointed at the little permit in the corner of my front left window, sat back and defiantly looked at him as if to say "Let me see you not turn your idle ass around and shuffle back into that box, press that little button and lift this gate."

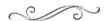

I missed the comforting smell of the *Brötchen* and coffee. Though I was never hungry, the familiar smell always reassured me. Let me know I was temporarily, at least, at home.

Marc would still be sleeping when I arrived. The nurses knew that I would be there at the break of day and that I alone wanted to care for him. After sleeping several hours I wanted him to wake up to me. They would bring a fresh change of clothes, a small stack of washcloths, a couple of towels. An ample supply of *Penaten* baby cream, lotion, powder, liquid soap, shampoo, green boxes of tissues, a thermometer and a spray bottle of disinfectant were staples on our little table. First came delightful snuggling, then I had to take his temperature. Aside from a doctor or nurse occasionally stopping by and lifting an eyebrow, we really weren't disturbed throughout our long, long day.

When Helmut came up in the evenings I let him give Marc his bottle while I told him about our day. One looked down while the other looked up not quite sure what to make of the other. The scene was beautiful, but there was something wrong with the picture.

Marc was thriving, yet his oxygen values remained dangerously low.

CHAPTER TEN

Change and Acceptance

Unbelievable things were happening. Things I wouldn't find out about until years later.

Ever since the unexplainable swelling had subsided, I had been at odds with the nonbelievers. So it was Helmut who did all the negotiating, ping-ponging back and forth between me and the Professor. I wanted Marc to have surgery. How long did they actually expect me to remain caged in this hospital surrounded by an impassive folk gawking at me, anticipating the moment fate would fall like a guillotine and forever sever the bond between me and my child?

We'd been cooped up here 'waiting' in this place day in and day out for nearly two months and our baby wasn't dying. The whole approach to this situation was sick. Get up every day, go nurture your baby and wait for him to die. What is that? For weeks? Don't think anguish had forced me into delusion. No, no, no, no, no. The bottom line of the prognosis was clear to me. It's just that rigor mortis had stiffened the perspective of those around me, but I didn't live in that world. I had to give God a hand in this miracle. In my mind it didn't take a rocket scientist to see that if this child didn't get adequate oxygen, and soon, he could very well end up brain damaged on top of everything else. I had no idea if my thoughts were right or wrong, but I didn't care because that was my gut feeling and I stood my ground. Helmut spoke with the Professor. He couldn't be swayed. I didn't relent. This went on and on. For days.

Despite the Professor's knowledge, skill and experience, deep in his heart I don't think Helmut believed Marc was going anywhere. But he was afraid. It stands to reason that because he had watched his mother very slowly and painfully die from cancer a year before Marc's birth, a strong aversion to seeing his son suffer restrained his enthusiasm for surgery. He had nothing else to go on. No one had offered him a dose of optimism. Though Marc wasn't acting out of the ordinary, call it mother's intuition, I could feel the clock ticking. No, make that a bomb.

"Helmut," I said as we hovered over Marc one day, "if we don't do something after all this time he's been staying alive and he dies because we didn't help him, how are you going to live with that? How do you expect me to? The fainthearted will always be fainthearted. They reap no rewards, not in this life and not in the one hereafter. And that scares me to death. We've got to at least try."

He could feel the ticking too.

In the meantime, unbeknownst to me, a miracle worker, by the name of Dr. Aldo Castañeda, former surgeon-in-chief at Children's Hospital Boston and William E. Ladd Professor of Child Surgery at Harvard Medical School, who is perhaps best known for establishing the benefits of repairing congenital heart defects at the earliest possible age, had tried to intervene.

Mama had found Dr. Castañeda in Boston and spoke with him on the phone. This gracious man took the time to call the clinic and spoke with the *Oberärtztin*, the woman doctor who was assistant medical director of children's cardiology. The Professor was away for a seminar and she was in charge during his brief absence. When he returned, she told him of Dr. Castañeda's call in which he implored them to operate, to perform a procedure that would buy time. I never knew of the call until many, many years later.

They mimicked him. "Aldo called," they sing-songed and snickered amongst themselves. "...and the mother," the Professor remarked, "is *'unbelehrbar'*" (obstinate). I guess he assumed that I just couldn't get it through my thick skull to give up on my baby.

That's what I can't fit in my mind.

Meanwhile, Dr. Gillor had set off on his own journey. He wasn't sure what should or shouldn't be done, but he'd heard the venerated name Castañeda and thought if Dr. Castañeda thought we should operate, well, maybe there might be something to it. That, along with the fact that Marc was growing and, also having observed me battling the elements for two months spurred him on.

The surgeon who would perform the surgery, was also the director of heart surgery at this institution. Dr. Gillor hadn't intended to pull him out of his meeting. He didn't even know he was in a meeting.

"Listen," Dr. Gillor said. "The parents of Marc Mayer want to operate, they want to make a shunt." The surgeon was furious.

"You pulled me out of a meeting just to tell me the parents have changed their minds?" he said.

"Well, it's quite urgent. If the ductus closes the child will die. It is astounding that after such a long time it is still open and it is possible that it could close any minute," Dr. Gillor said.

"Well, I'm not going to give you an immediate date for surgery just because the parents have changed their minds!" he said.

"So what shall we tell the parents?" Dr. Gillor said.

"Tell them what you want. But I will not operate within the next two weeks."

Several days later, the Professor told us that there were only two operating theaters available and one of them was not in working order and because of the scheduled operations for the other babies, we would have to wait at least three weeks. To hell with that. We couldn't wait another minute.

Frantic, on February 1, 1985, I flew out of Cologne at one thirty in the afternoon headed towards London's Brompton Hospital carrying a copy of Marc's cineangiocardiogram, his medical report and The Lord's Prayer. Family in Seattle had found out about a children's cardiothoracic surgeon, Dr. Christopher Lincoln, who maybe, just maybe could help us.

Helmut was waiting for me when I stepped off the plane back in Cologne. The moment our eyes met, he knew. After assuring me that Marc was fine, I told him what had happened the last five hours. We rode to the hospital in silence. The kind of silence that says everything.

It was way after midnight. I had just come home from the clinic, tired and deeply depressed with my results in England that afternoon, frustrated and feeling so very sorry for myself. All I wanted was to have my baby. Why did it have to be so difficult?

I remember answering the telephone in the basement. I don't recall why I was down there; it's not as if I had any luggage to store away. The phone was the same dull olive green as the tissue boxes in the hospital. I had never seen such an ugly color on a telephone. At the time, it was not uncommon here. I snatched the phone from the receiver on the first ring.

"Hello?"

"Tracie, it's Mommy, honey. How's Marc?"

Everyone was in the kitchen, huddled around the speakerphone. My sisters and Daddy chipped in all at once, "What happened in London? What did the doctor say? How did things go?"

They were all so worried about Marc and me. They knew I was at the end of my rope, not sure if I could hang on another few weeks waiting for surgery let alone worrying about the surgery itself and if Marc's oxygen would drop down to nearly nothing in that space of time or if his ductus would close or if he'd start swelling again. So many things could go wrong.

"Well," I sighed. "The doctor had a variation on the theme, but really didn't differ in opinion too much from the doctors here." That was it in the nutshell. But he had been kind and patient and had the friendliest secretary. Beverly was her name. I remember her offering me a cup of tea. "Would you like it white or black," she asked me. It took me a second. White or black? Cream! She must mean cream. "Black," I said taking a seat. Tea. Black or white. I'd never heard that before. Cobwebs in my head kept me entangled those days.

"Tracie, Tracie honey, there's a doctor in Düsseldorf. Isn't that over there by you?"

"Yes, Mama, it's only about a half-hour drive from here," I said as I cradled the telephone receiver in the crook of my neck while I searched the desk, pulling out drawers looking for paper and pen.

"The doctor's name is Bourgeois. Professor Maurice Bourgeois. He's supposed to be a good doctor for babies with my grandbaby's illness."

"Sugar?"

"Daddy?" I rested my head against the palm of my hand; delicate teardrops stung the folds of my eyes. I was again daring myself to look towards that rainbow.

"Now you listen to your daddy carefully. You remember Woody Woodhouse?"

"Sure I do," I said.

When Woody Woodhouse and his wife arrived in Seattle from Detroit I was just a little bit more than a notion. Daddy rented them an apartment while they were getting on their feet and Woody ended up singing in Daddy's combo. Over the years, as each pursued his own purpose in life, Woody found himself taking on employment at the University of Washington hospital. Their friendship had remained solid for over thirty years.

"Well, Woody is the one who gave us the information. This doctor is supposed to be the man. You get him on the phone first thing when you wake up in the morning and make arrangements to get my grandson over there to him."

"I'll be on it first thing, Daddy," I said.

He hesitated. "You stay tough now. Marc's counting on you, we all are. Everything's gonna be alright. You listen to your daddy. And remember, ain't no givin' up and no givin' out."

"Okay Daddy... I know, I know. I'll call you guys tomorrow and let you know what happened. Just keep praying, everybody. Just ask everybody to pray."

"We will Trace, darlin', sugar," they all pitched in. "We love you. Get some rest."

"I love you all too," I said.

I had just laid my head on my pillow, willing myself to jettison all stumbling blocks from my mind, when it dawned on me: tomorrow was Saturday.

I cursed the darkness.

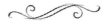

Professor Bourgeois's heavily accented English bridging the telephone wires that fourth of February Monday morning felt like a sedative being pumped into my veins.

Two days after my speaking with Professor Bourgeois and nearly a week since Dr. Gillor had incurred the wrath of the surgeon, Marc was admitted to the University Clinic in Düsseldorf in preparation for surgery under the care of cardiologist Professor Bourgeois. The surgery itself would be carried out by Professor Bircks the day after, on February 7, 1985.

We hadn't 'changed' our minds. We just didn't accept their minds anymore.

CHAPTER ELEVEN

Why Do You Cry?

The operation went without complication. Professor Bircks performed a left-sided Blalock-Taussig shunt so named after the two pioneering doctors who developed the operation.

Dr. Helen Brooke Taussig is recognized as the first lady of pediatric cardiology in the world. She'd read that the ductus arteriosis had been surgically closed and theorized that if an artery to the heart could be closed, one could also be opened, thereby helping children with congenital heart defects who were blue because they weren't receiving enough oxygen in their blood. She approached Dr. Blalock with her theory. Dr. Alfred Blalock had been working with the black cardiac pioneer Vivian Thomas. It was actually Mr. Thomas who developed the surgical techniques used in treating these "blue" or cyanotic babies. The first operation was carried out in 1944. Beginning as an assistant to Dr. Blalock, the complex partnership between these two men lasted thirty-four years and inspired the 2004 film *Something the Lord Made.*

Time stood still as minutes ticked by in the operating theater. That apprehensive feeling of hanging on by a thread had woven itself into a blanket of cautious calm and had settled itself around me. We were far from out of the woods, but for the very first time, I felt like I wasn't looking down a tunnel of darkness that faded into black. Now I could see a flicker of light at the end.

Though the operation was complication free, the post-operative course was made difficult due to bronchial pneumonia. Nine days after the surgery Marc was taken off artificial respiration and the final extubation was carried out several days later. Once all the tubes had been removed, I was allowed to feed him a bottle. His oxygen saturation post-op was around seventy percent. Taking all into consideration, this palliative operation had been a success.

I was on my way to Marc one day shortly after his surgery when the telephone stopped me in my tracks. Concerned because his desire to eat was sporadic, my first thought was that it was the hospital calling.

"Hello?"

It was my gynecologist's office. The receptionist connected me with the doctor.

"How are you?" he asked. "How is Marc?"

"Okay, everything is fine," I told him.

Even if things weren't exactly rosy, there was no point moaning to him about it. And I had to get a move on. Though I'd been driving to Düsseldorf every day for three weeks, there was always the possibility that my mind, constantly shuttling between retrospect and anticipation, wouldn't be attentive to my location on the road before me and I would drive past or take the wrong *Ausfahrt* (exit) from the Autobahn.

Either way, this could end up being catastrophic as it isn't always possible to take an exit off the highway and loop around to rejoin the motorway. You must drive to the next village, stop, ask, understand, hope that whoever is helping you is not just being kind and guessing which direction to send you, and set off again in what could be a completely different direction. God forbid heavy traffic. This happened to me twice; the second time I vowed it would never happen again.

After flying along at the utmost speed I suddenly realized that I was not seeing anything recognizable. The turbulence that made my nervous system feel like it was trapped in an air pocket began the second I realized that I couldn't remember how far back it had been since I'd seen something recognizable. Follow the sign towards the *Innenstadt* (city center), I knew I must've done that. And at the airport sign bear left...Did I? Continue straight until the old town and then...I gasped. Without warning they began popping up to the left of me on the opposite side of the motorway, first one and then another: windmills. I was headed towards Holland. Never again. He really had to hurry up and say what he had to say.

"The results of your pap smear from last week are back," he said. "I'm concerned because there appear to be some cell changes."

"What kind of cell changes?" I asked, easing myself down onto the couch.

"This is an abnormal changing, dysplasia, it is called. It is not now cancer but I'm afraid if we do nothing the lesions could turn cancerous."

"So how long would it take for that to happen?" I asked him.

"Your numbers stand between 3d and 4a. Five is cancer. The sooner we take care of this the better."

"So what has to be done?" I asked him.

"You'll have to go into the hospital."

"What? Can't they do whatever they've got to do on an outpatient basis? I've got to be at the hospital with Marc."

"No, unfortunately not," he said. "You will have to check in for a few days. The surgeon will perform a conization. It is surgery and you will have to stay in the hospital for a couple days."

I tried to make Plan B spring into my mind. There wasn't one.

"Okay, look. Can you make the arrangements for me? The only clinic I'll go to is the one in Düsseldorf."

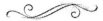

The surgeon tried to comfort me as I lay prepped for surgery. He stroked my face, looked at me questioningly. "Why do you cry? You don't have to cry," he said. Marc hadn't taken his bottle so well again that morning. "My baby, my baby," I said turning my head away from him. And then it was dark.

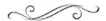

The surgeon had instructed his staff to make me stay in bed that first day, but the day after my surgery, I was strong enough to waddle over to the building where Marc lay. At eight o'clock that morning I got the whole feeding down him, ninety-five milliliters, just a little over three ounces in twenty-five minutes.

Fortunately everything was fine with me and two days later I was released from the hospital and four days after that, thirty-seven days after his surgery, and one hundred and six days subsequent to his birth, I could finally bundle up our son and Helmut could drive us home.

I remember standing at the door of his office, holding Marc in my arms, getting the last words of encouragement and direction from Professor Bourgeois. Marc was to take medicine twice a day, eat roughly every four hours whereby I should keep track of how long it took him to eat how much, check how often he made a stool, be observant of any changes in it, and weigh him daily.

Monitoring the weight of his nutritional intake and comparing it with his body weight would help me detect any unusual weight increase which could mean a buildup of fluid somewhere. We were also instructed to visit him in two weeks. Thereafter we could continue our checkups back at the University Clinic in Cologne.

It could have been that I had asked the same question twice but in a different format or maybe I was just doing the 'double-check' or maybe it was an 'in the event that happens what shall I do' question, but Helmut tried to cut me off, enough with the questions already. Without uttering a word, Professor Bourgeois turned his head towards him, knitted his brow and narrowed his eyes into slits shutting him up and without blinking directed his reopened gaze towards me and slowly nodded, indicating I should carry on with my questions until I felt comfortable that I had everything down just right.

Yes!

We bought a baby scale on the way home. After we got settled in, Helmut drew up a chart with eight columns. The first column had the day of the month and 8:00 for 8 A.M. It began with the 16th of March. The next four columns noted the amount of milliliters of milk/amount of time to eat and the times 12:00, 16:00, 20:00 and 24:00. The next column, quite narrow when compared to the others, was only wide enough for a *Ja* (yes) or *Nein* (no) for stool and the final column said *sonstiges* (anything else).

It seemed like it had been forever since the first moment Marc had seen the light of day. Though I was physically exhausted from being tied up in knots for so long and my weight had whittled down to less than my pre-pregnancy weight, I felt re-born. That first day home the only regret I had was that I couldn't breast-feed our son. I didn't even remember when the last drop of liquid gold had fallen from my bosom.

Pity.

That night when I put him to bed, his room finally felt right. I turned the little knob of the mobile fastened to the railings of his bed. Pastel-colored lambs and ponies twirled in time to the lulling music above him.

When I laid my head down on my pillow that night, a heavy sigh escaped my soul. I had finally, finally risen to the water's surface and could take a breath again.

An inextinguishable frenzy had been quelled by a tranquility as uncrumpled as the velvety green flow of rolling hills.

I smiled.

We made it!

CHAPTER TWELVE

Life is Wonderful

Finally nestled in our sanctuary, I just wanted to bolt the door and raise the drawbridge.

That was not meant to be.

Too few – four, to be exact – joyous days after our liberation from the hospital shackles, I found myself slowly driving down Main Street, a one-way thoroughfare in Frechen, a little village no more than twenty minutes from our home. My eyes, by turns, darted away from the road ahead to Marc strapped in the carry car seat in the rearview mirror, to the flat-roofed buildings lining the sidewalk. I was searching for building number 19-21. Or was it two buildings? I didn't think to ask that.

Tardiness wasn't trendy in my book and as you may have guessed by now I had developed an absolute rabid aversion to finding myself lost, so though we weren't late, it felt as if all my pores had opened, urgently willing the building or buildings to appear before my eyes. In spite of this, apprehension descended spread-eagle upon me. The closer I sensed we were to our impending destination, the more difficult it became to draw a deep breath of air. I felt surefooted on a banana peel.

I envisioned Mama in the passenger seat reassuring me, could almost feel her.

"God never gives us more than we can bear. Everything will be alright." That's what she would say. Nonetheless, I couldn't pry either hand away from my two fisted lock on the steering wheel.

"I am so sick of doctors and needles, I could scream! If I ever see either again it would be too soon. So why are we here? Must this be? Am I a glutton for punishment? And why so soon? We just got home – what if he spots something and sends us back to the hospital? I'm not going back to the hospital. I don't give a damn what he says."

"Tracie, no tirades," I said to myself. "Don't forget our promise now. You know we decided that we would bridge over, not plunge into the depths of worry waterways. Everything's fine. No one is going to send you back to the hospital. And stop acting like a two-year-old. Stomping your feet won't change the fact that Marc has to get his polio, diphtheria and tetanus immunizations; he's a month late as it is. These are serious diseases, killers and cripplers of children. Be thankful he's here to even get the shots. Every baby gets them, or at least should get them, so let us not rue the routine. Compared to everything else that's happened up till now, you'll handle this with your eyes shut. Don't fret."

Yeah, right. Don't fret. My insides curdled. I dreaded the possibility of being thrown back into the lion's den;

no guardrails and unfamiliar. So extremely sobering. I couldn't help but be on the lookout, a wary eye on the outlook. To circumvent letdown, the only expectation I had was of myself; no matter what, I would not waver. I was right. After all I'd been through, I felt certain I could count on that. And a box of tissues.

As I recall, Dr. Gillor recommended Dr. Tinschman to me. From what he knew, he was a nice man and good pediatrician, treated children with cardiovascular disease and his office, though not exactly a stone's throw away, was easily accessible for me by car. Okay, we'll see, I remember thinking. What I really meant was, Lord, please give me a break.

The car edged along the street. Good thing it wasn't a heavily trafficked area. I crept along, my eyes squinting at the numbers on the buildings to the right of me. No pressing need to consider the buildings on the left side of the street, they were all even numbered. Double-check anyway. A paint store monopolized a good portion of that block – upon which, by the way, I could see no number. Contiguous to the paint store was a dance studio, linked by a pub, a kiosk, and then a flower shop. So what I was looking for was definitely not on this side of the street. Put it away.

I stalled at the corner in front of the paint store. The thoroughfare had come to an abrupt end. The culprit here, there and everywhere in front of my nose thwarted any and all hope of driving further down Main Street. Automobiles were banned, barred, verboten in the *Fußgänger* (Pedestrian) zone. The length of each side of it appeared to be measured in miles. It was a virtual cobblestoned colony teeming with retail and grocery stores, potted outdoor plants, banks, bakeries, butcher shops, cafes, old people, young people, strolling, pushing carriages, riding bikes as far as the eye could see...eventually dots in the distance.

"Where is the building?" I said out loud. "It has to be here."

If I continued on this street following its curve around the corner it would no longer be Main Street. I needed Main Street, damn it! Main Street 19-21.

"I know I followed Helmut's directions to a T. I must have passed it," I said to myself again out loud. This was one of the perks about having my baby in the car, or at least I thought it was. I could talk out loud and passersby would assume I was chatting away with him. I recall thinking I should smile in case someone was really looking. I put the car in reverse and slowly backed up, waving the two oncoming cars behind to drive around me.

The office was indeed just seconds behind me, on the right side of the street, sandwiched between a kitchenware store and a boutique. Though the entrance was neither visible nor accessible from the street, 19-21 was posted on the building. There was still space in front of the paint store. I pulled up in front of its big display window, shoved the gearshift to park, opened the door, jumped out, locked the doors and ran across the street towards the sign: *Kinderärtze* (Pediatricians). This was the place, but where the hell is the entrance, I asked myself as I desperately searched for a 'go that way' arrow in between the signs written in gobbledygook. I saw a narrow passageway behind two glass doors with the same sign. "The entrance must be beyond those doors," I concluded. "There's no place else it could possibly be." So I scooted back across the street, hopped in the car, pulled the key from the starter and grabbed my purse. Jogging around to the opposite rear side of the car, I swung the door open, unfastened the belt and lifted Marc from his car seat.

The elevator lifted us smoothly to the second floor, its doors sliding open directly outside the office. *Kinderärzte*. The door was slightly ajar.

I stepped inside, gave our names at the front desk: Tracie and Marc Mayer. Maybe it was because I introduced us with both our given names (as far as I was concerned, the umbilical cord had not been severed from my maternal blood vessel, this was therefore a collective appointment), and I anyway wasn't yet used to saying Frau Mayer, or maybe I just looked like a first-time mom, or a first-time mom foreigner who couldn't speak German, or...whatever, one of the assistants heeded my sense of unfamiliarity and as she spoke, kindly turned and pointed us in the direction of the nearest waiting area.

Settling into the only empty chair, I glanced at my watch: we were on time! We even had a couple minutes to spare. Time enough for me to get my thoughts together. Thank goodness.

"Punctuality always makes a good impression. Maybe since we were conscientious enough to be on time, he won't find anything wrong and send us back to the hospital."

"Tracie, stop it!" I said.

"Okay, okay, okay!" I said, bracing myself.

Soft-spoken, sturdy, sure of himself and what he was doing, Dr. Tinschman smoothed the wrinkle right out of my brow. And he did it in pretty darn good English! Taking Marc from my arms he lifted him in the air, smiled up at him and said, "Hello, little man. Life is wonderful and it will be for you too." Now THAT'S what I was talkin' about!

This stranger boosted my morale like a satellite soaring towards the moon. Support up till now had been scarce to say the least and though I was buoyed by a steady stream of words of encouragement and prayers from my family and friends in America, they were all still across the ocean, a world away.

Firmly entrenched in the belief that how I interacted with Marc would play a major role in his survival, I had decided to keep all negativity away from me. People included. I reasoned that if my global view was always clouded with teardrops, I would not number among my possessions the serene yet certain vision to instill in my son the necessary provisions for a well-stocked spirit, one that stirred his body and soul to sound the trumpet and revel in the festivity of life.

Moping and woe is me could not, would not and should not be a part of the program if I was to succeed. Bearing up under the weight of it all required granitic strength, especially the subduing of my anxiousness, but this was not about Tracie. Someone had moved the goalposts, but that did not diminish my responsibility to ensure my son that he had been entrusted to able hands, that he was indeed a child of fortune. So it was crucial for me as well as Marc that his primary health caretaker not be bogged down with a murky mind-set. And it turns out that this doctor holding my son in his hands had team spirit! And it took no coaxing from me! Hallelujah!

Silently expressing thanks to God for our good fortune while staying deeply engrossed in conversation, closely observing how he turned Marc's baby body this way and that as he examined him, I was untroubled by the jarring alarm that pierced holes through the air every couple of seconds. I mean, for all I knew, that was just a part of the backdrop on Main Street Frechen.

"So it's normal when—"

The door to the examination room burst open cutting me off. One of his assistants excitedly jabbered something to him. He looked away from Marc towards her and jabbered something back. She again to him. He cooed with Marc a moment and then he lifted his eyes towards me. "Mrs. Mayer," he said. "Are you by chance driving an Audi Quattro?"

I got gooseflesh.

"Red?" I asked him.

"Red," he said, suppressing a chuckle.

"Why?" I said, catapulting over to the window. I looked down at the street and caught my breath. The screaming whistle was coming from the mile-long red and white *Straßenbahn* (tram) whose wheels coursed steel rails uninterruptedly from Frechen to the heart of Cologne...thatmycarwasblocking!

Wishful thinking could not banish my embarrassment nor make the tram stop its window-shattering shrieking. I darted away from the window and snatched the keys from my purse. Shooting a glance his way, I saw Dr. Tinschman dandling Marc, smiling at me as if to say over the years he'd seen a lot, this was really no big deal, though I was sure it was near the top of his "this is the stupidest thing I've ever witnessed" list. I didn't utter a word but if I had, it would have been, "I'll be right back! You'd better not drop my baby."

The dozen of adjudicating "We know where we are and where to park" eyes that fixed upon me as I tore out of the office felt like incendiary bombs stoking 98.6 F. (37 C.) into an all-out hot flash. Down to my very quick. How could I be so stupid? Damn!

I didn't wait on the elevator.

"See? Parking in the wrong place! That's what you get for having a nervous feather in your ass," I said.

"Oh shut up and help me figure out where I can park as close as possible as fast as I can!"

I purposely avoided looking at the driver. I wanted to profusely apologize and ask him to please understand that this was my first time here in Frechen and it had been stressful looking for the doctor's office and though overcome with relief that I'd found it, over the past months I'd developed the collywobbles about all matters medical and truly didn't want to be here, and I swear that I had no idea that I'd parked over tram tracks, I would normally never do such a stupid thing, after all I'd been driving since I was sixteen years old and knew how to drive and properly parallel park, but I couldn't jabber my thoughts and was just so thankful for the lull in the air, I yanked the car door open, jumped in, twisted the key in the ignition switch, jerked the gear lever into reverse and looking over my right shoulder out the rear window had the luck to find a parking space on the correct side of the street just a breath away from the entrance. I sprinted back up the stairs to his office. He hadn't dropped him.

The universe could be merciful.

CHAPTER THIRTEEN

Holding Steady

So March eased into April. Developing taste buds stimulated by the unfamiliar flavors of pureed fresh fruits, vegetables and porridge were supped up thimbleful after thimbleful. Far from having a voracious appetite, Marc ate as though it was really a matter of taste. As a result, his weight bobbed up and down in its steady ascent. A breezy, but cloudless day gave us the opportunity to enjoy our first leisurely stroll to our neighborhood shopping mall. Marc was snuggly tucked underneath a puff of blanket bulging from his *Kinderwagen.*

Well-meaning excursionists had no hesitation stopping me to get a peek inside the pram.

"Ist er nicht lecker?" one after another they cooed, alternately smiling down at Marc and then up at me and back to him. I returned their smiles with a proud motherly smile. That was about all I could bring to the table. Judging from the way they curiously peered at me, it was unlikely they expected more. I appreciated their apparent kindnesses and though never intending to be rude, had to several times put the wheels of the

pram in motion as I really didn't like these complete strangers exhaling their oohs and aahhs all over my baby. Any longer than fifteen seconds overtaxed me anyway as invariably their cordial congratulations picked up momentum and rolled on into cryptic chatter.

That evening as we three lay cuddled in our bed I asked Helmut, "Sweetie, what does *'er ist lecker'* mean?"

Memorized to the best of my ability, I knew I didn't regurgitate it the way it actually was pronounced, but was sure since I'd heard it so often throughout the course of our afternoon, that it must be a common German expression Helmut would be familiar with. I had it close enough. His eyes twinkled.

"Did somebody say that to you today?"

"Oh, my goodness! Lots of times. Every time somebody looked at Marc in his stroller. You should have seen him, he was so cute, each time someone smiled at him, he smiled back. I couldn't believe it."

"Ist er nicht lecker?" means *'ist er nicht süß?'"*

I looked at him, waiting.

"I'm still not there yet, Helmut."

He burst out laughing.

"In English it probably means 'isn't he sweet.'"

Aha! That's what I thought. Well-wishers peeking in the pram, taking delight in our eye candy.

A cocoon of contentment had enveloped our little family. We pulled up the blankets, played footsies and quickly entangled our arms and legs. Angel in the middle. A true love knot. Now this was heaven...

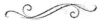

That third Friday in April smelled like any other morning: aftershave, baby powder, coffee, formula, just unplugged hair curlers, and butter melting on toast. The sun had inhaled and hung swollen bright in the blue sky over the Rhine River, promising a glorious day.

Marc sucked four ounces of formula from his bottle and then he neither ate nor drank anything else. Not at midmorning. Not at noon. Not in the afternoon. Not at all. Period.

By the time daylight had begun to slip away, leaving a hint of dusk on the horizon, I was deep in the throes of panic. No-way-out deep. He wasn't cranky or constipated, wet or too warm, he slept as he saw fit, there were no signs of trouble or distress that I could see, and on a grand scale of one to ten, that rated minus five. What did I know about all the reasons why a baby would have no appetite? Was this just a normal baby thing or...?

Asking Helmut would have just amounted to taking a shortcut back to my nebulous point of departure and only cause him extra worry. With him putting all his energies into getting the business off the ground, and me being a stay-at-home mother, I didn't want to unnecessarily load him down with the particulars of what I considered to be my domain anyway, just as he didn't burden me with all the headaches of his making a living for us.

To this extent, in supporting ourselves, we supported each other. With both of our cups filled to overflowing, he and I found tremendous comfort in knowing one could unfailingly depend upon the other and that each of us, no matter what the circumstance, would give his best when rising to the occasion. Our oneness evolved from the sum of our complementary parts. This unspoken interconnection spoke the truth to the natural affinity we felt for one another. Shaped by our passionate love, together we were indistinguishable. Kindred spirits since that day on the beach in Vallarta. We were blessed.

I thought it would last forever.

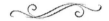

By nightfall, Marc still hadn't eaten and I hadn't been able to worry hunger into him. I placed a call to Dr. Tinschman.

He set his black leather bag on the dressing table in Marc's room next to the satin-clad rosy- cheeked jester supporting a lamp, pulled out his stethoscope, and then warmed it in his hands before gently pressing it here and there along the surface of Marc's body. He listened, touched and observed, sometimes with a squint. My anxious eyes scrutinizing his features didn't hinder his ease with the examination which was a good thing because my gaze held steady. If he was going to say "Uh-oh," I wanted to read it on his face before he said it. The Greek philosopher Heraclitus must have had me, the resident alien in mind, when he said that the: "Eyes are more accurate witnesses than ears." I had grown accustomed over the last months to putting more faith in what I saw than in what I heard. Things would stay that way as long as I could neither make head nor tail of the language. Secretly I felt: stare hard at his face. Stare hard and defy his mouth to utter the unthinkable.

Before he left, he assured us that he detected no danger signals. Marc's appetite would surely pick up by tomorrow. Don't worry, be patient. There was really nothing I could do but keep an eye on him, check his temperature, attempt periodically to get something down him, and last but not least, try to calm my nerves and not proceed to go slowly stark raving mad because he was after all a baby, a real-life human being who would eat and drink according to his own plan. He was not a doll designed to please me with a mechanism that when wound would waken saucer eyes with a flutter that would then blink blink blink while a rosebud mouth opened and closed in tempo to the tick-tick-ticking of an unwinding key.

My tension ebbed the following morning when a warm bottle triggered Marc's rooting reflex. Throughout the course of the day, his appetite picked up. In spurts.

May 1: The right side of his face appeared swollen. Slightly, just to the point where I was sure of it. Or was it my imagination?

May 30: The second day of a phlegmy cough as well as an occasional slight trembling while crying sent us to Dr. Tinschman's office. A cough syrup and sedative soothed the both of us.

June 10: Another cold. Another syrup to reduce infection and feeling of malaise.

June 13: For the very first time while lying on his stomach, Marc raised his head and held it up! As I watched him, my spirit, heretofore violated by his limitations, leaped towards the heavens. He was steadily gaining weight and thoroughly enjoyed another newfound ability: amusing himself by making noises with his mouth. Helmut and I were tickled pink!

June 27: Warm to the touch, too warm, runny nose.

5:15 P.M. Coughing and temperature an elevated 38 Celsius.

7:00 P.M. Temperature 38.5 C.

7:35 P.M. Stethoscope, the scrutinized face deep in thought. The jester, faintly smiling, emitted a soft light over the opened neck of the leather bag.

Penicillin.

Panacea.

Please.

9:30 P.M. 38.2 C.

11:00 P.M. 37.8 C.

In the darkness of his room, I quietly reached over the mahogany vertical slats of his crib, folded back the blanket and rested my palm on his back. Flat, unheaving. Almost still.

Then, his breath soft whispers against my fingers.

3:10 A.M. Forehead, neck, cheeks no longer kindled.

The antidote had destroyed the adversary.

Safe.

Silence.

Sleep...except for my senses. They wouldn't shut down.

Nothing had changed in the room. The only notable difference this time around was that rather than feeling my heart thumping with fear, my chest was swollen with pride July 3rd at our first checkup. I boasted to the Professor that Marc was a really happy baby, slept well and had gained seven pounds since his birth. He was now reaching and touching and holding and just loved shaking his silver rattle, one of a slew of gifts from Grandma and Grandpa in America.

Because the swelling had subsided after a day or two, I found no need to mention it. Basically, aside from the minor coughing and the infection that was cleared up by the antibiotics, and a stuffy nose for which he'd been taking nose drops intermittently over the past two days, we hadn't had any significant difficulties I told him. He almost smiled. I think.

I held Marc close, kissing him gently as the needle pierced his finger. Though the Professor sprayed a numbing agent on the point of puncture beforehand, Marc nonetheless let out a wail that testified to the elasticity of his lungs. The results of the laboratory work would, amongst other values, reveal the amount of oxygen in his blood. Ninety to one hundred percent is ideal, however, in our imperfect world, one can indeed live with less and lead a normal or nearly normal life. The rest of the examination, including a one-and-two dimensional echocardiogram, hadn't revealed any reason to give cause for alarm so we were free to go. He told me to call the following day for the results of the blood test.

Bouncing from the last step of the staircase onto the main floor with my blanketed bundle snuggled to my breast, I nearly skipped out the automated doors. The absolute euphoric feeling of wellness was like an old friend by my side; a reassurance that yes (!), the center of the universe was holding steady. Inhale relief. Deeply. Breathe out anxiety till my stomach crunched. I reveled in it. My psyche effervesced. If I didn't get to Helmut soon, I would surely pop, just go right ahead and burst into one zillion ecstatic pieces. Certain we were over the hump, I dared to toss worry to the dust heap and whoop it up!

CHAPTER FOURTEEN

Trials and Tribulations, Twists and Tricks

"His oxygen level is only 49.5%," the Professor said the next morning.

I went limp.

"I want you to continue giving him his medication and come back to me in four weeks for his next checkup. If the oxygen level remains low, it will be necessary to plan the next heart catheter examination."

Baffled and barely breathing, I don't remember him saying good-bye. My hand stuttered as I noted the appointment down in the calendar, all the while my other hand clutched the receiver to my ear, holding on as if to a lifeline. Was that it? Couldn't be.

I was still waiting to hear that I shouldn't worry, that this was just a precautionary measure; in the complex system of the human body values go up and down every day, and sometimes low oxygen values appear after the kind of surgery Marc had, particularly in babies, because certain physiological processes are very hard at work coordinating themselves, maybe even the stuffy nose had something to do with it, but it doesn't matter because in any event, all these cells and atoms are learning to adjust to life outside the womb, and it can take some time before everything fits into place. But don't worry, things will fit into place.

The line had been disengaged, and the dial tone droned in my ear. I slowly replaced the receiver to the cradle.

Dropping onto the couch I closed my eyes. God Almighty...I'd done all I could and I felt so powerless. A welter of emotions, primarily a searing anger at the injustice of it all, overtook me. We'd come so far and we still hadn't come far enough and I was afraid of all the unknowns lying in wait, and just how many of these pricks and probes and surgical procedures my baby could endure. The moment was one of pure disbelief. I didn't want sugarplums, just an affirmation – and not one scrawled in invisible ink – of a future where all would be well. Was that too much to ask for? Was it?

Marc's cry charged the air, drawing me out of the grotto of my mind. It was a declaration that I'd best discard the notion of a perfectly predictable life and had better start enjoying every minute of the present because it – the here and now – is the only thing truly available. The only thing. At our fingertips. This moment. And it is fleeting.

The tests showed his levels to be at 55%. A reprieve.

Two weeks later 53%. I was instructed to give him iron as a prophylactic to stimulate the production of more red blood cells whose duty is to carry oxygen throughout the body. These baby- sized microorganisms can, particularly if oxygen deficient, have a tendency to clump together causing a hiatus in their rhythm of continuous flow; thrombosis it is called. How could such tiny little things create such a great big problem?

The following Sunday he slept till noon. Woke up fussy and slept some more. Never slept so much. I thought that maybe it was too hot outside. Wondered if the heat could make the blood thicker. If it could, would that make him unusually tired? Couldn't find a reason for his crankiness. Once again, a shroud of questions began to unfold, veiling me in confusion.

A puncture of the right artery set the stage for the heart catheterization one month later. After three days in the hospital, we returned home September 12. Contrary to the previous low values, the oxygen saturation of his blood was between 68 and 72 percent. But the value of the hemoglobin, a protein found in the red blood cells, was too high, and in the previous weeks had been steadily climbing. Marc's delayed motor development, due to his physical weakness, substantiated this and was a strong indicator that another operation would be necessary.

The Professor had conferred with the surgeon. The same surgeon who refused to operate the first time. A right sided Blalock-Taussig shunt loomed on the December horizon.

October 8: Two upper teeth erupted. Every little thing about our baby was a thrill for Helmut and me. Most often we felt haunted on a high wire, but when he grinned those precious pearls at us, and we'd kiss his drool and smell his sweet breath, it gave us such joy that we'd momentarily forget how fragile the thread of life is and jump into the sunshine of parenthood headfirst, as though we hadn't a problem in the world. Gray clouds be damned.

October 10, 4:00 P.M. Temperature was 37.6 C.
    4:48 P.M. 37.9.
    4:55 P.M. 38.2.
    Well, by now, as I'm sure you can imagine, I had a peace-of-mind stocked medicine cabinet. I wasn't sure, but I had a feeling that the elevated temperature stemmed from his emerging teeth. His little chin shined, slippery with drool. He wasn't particularly miserable, had no cough and his temperature wasn't too high, so I figured I'd go by guess and by God. I had to let a positive-thinking attitude guide me and learn not to be

intimidated by his heart disease; he was after all going to have fevers and colds and teeth, and now was as good a time as any to get a firmness of mind and not let every little thing send me cowering to the telephone. I desperately needed to build up my supply of courage, common sense and mother's instincts instruments.

Now, because his only symptom was a slightly elevated temperature, I thought that I would attempt to grapple alone with the situation. And you know? To be quite honest, there was another little motive urging me on. I really didn't want Dr. Tinschman to feel as if I'd become like the fever reducing suppository about to be removed from its foil encasing, and slipped into Marc's little behind. In other words: a pain in the butt.

5:30 P.M. 38 C.

6:40 P.M. 37.2.

8:08 P.M. 37.1.

8:57 P.M. 37.2.

10:30 P.M. 38.2.

No rest for the wicked.

Next morning, 8:00 A.M. 38.5.

9:15 A.M. 37.9.

Going.

Going.

Gone.

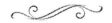

The 24th of October he vomited his beans and noodles. Diarrhea. A visit to our pediatrician again smoothed the wrinkle out of my brow.

November 3, he smooched with an opened mouth and clapped his hands when told to do so. In English.

His breathing was becoming noticeably heavy, not exactly laborious, but harder. Faster.

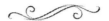

It was not a feeling of déjà vu I felt on the morning of December 5, 1985, as I watched a nurse wheel Marc in a glass box away from me headed toward the operating theater. Indeed, Marc's first operation had been just ten months ago. The only difference now was that we were at the clinic in Cologne.

I stood in the hallway of the ward. The smacking door opened, closed and they were gone. "Let go and let God," I could hear Mama say. Leaning against the wall for support, my feet gave way and I slid slowly down until I slumped to the floor, finally reaching my nadir. We had no cell phones then. There was no one to call anyway, with it being midnight in America.

Helmut was at work and would come as soon as he could. So I remained on the floor and I prayed, got lost in thought and prayed some more. Why didn't I get up? I don't know, maybe I just couldn't. Anyway, it really didn't matter. Floor, chair, inside, outside, up, down, every place was a place of torment. I really didn't know where else to go.

Immediately after the operation Marc was wheeled to the Intensive Care Unit. Four hours later he was taken off the respirator.

When I got home the very early hours of the following morning, I walked straight upstairs to the yellow and white dirty clothes hamper in his room. Lifted the lid and dropped it to the floor. I pulled out the last little jumpsuit he'd worn, held it to my face and breathed in his essence. I vowed not to wash any of his laundry until he came home.

The Pediatric Intensive Care Unit was white-light bright and smelled of antiseptics and disinfectants and babies and their wounds. Our son lay in a bed dwarfed by a labyrinth of tubes and gauze and adhesive strips. He was still off the respirator when I arrived several hours later.

I leaned over him and whispered a thousand times that he and I would survive this. Papa would too.

The next day, Saturday, due to respiratory insufficiency, he was re-intubated. The right-sided pleura drainage was filled with purulent fluid. Our son lay feverish.

It was late, nearing midnight. My eyes looked up and saw the Professor walking towards us.

"Good evening," he whispered.

"Hello, Professor, good evening," I said, regarding him from my chair.

He picked up the chart hanging from the foot of the bed and read it. Then he studiously observed Marc. All of a sudden his fist slammed against the bedposts. Stunned, a full moment lapsed before I could speak.

"What's the matter?" I said, unaware that his burst of emotion was provoked by the dismal fact that they were trying to kill off the infection with an antibiotical therapy consisting of three different kinds of medicine, none of which was working.

"Professor, what is the matter?"

It was as if I hadn't said a thing. He propped his elbow at an angle against the bed railings, brought his fist to his mouth and stared at Marc. Still as a statue.

His eyes remained riveted on our son when he finally told me it was late, that I should eat something, that I should go home.

He had to be kidding. Gingerly, I stood up from my chair and repeated the question, pausing after each word. Though not predetermined, I can't say if my actions were deliberate or not, no matter, he didn't go into details. He would try another constellation of chemicals to obliterate the bacteria immediately. He motioned for a nurse.

By Sunday nightfall, the pressure from the respiratory machine had been reduced down to five from a high of fifty. Monday, though its workings were still in his nose, Marc breathed on his own. The fever finally broke and on the following Sunday, the third Advent, the respirator was removed.

It was just this side of dusk Tuesday as Marc lay sleeping that I let my attentions wander, probably inspired by the fact that the inhalation device had been removed. One less machine. One less tube. One less bit of discomfort. One step closer to home.

Looking around the illuminated room my eyes fell upon baby after baby, and no one standing by to urge him or her to fight the good fight. So I took the liberty to make good use of my time while my son rested.

I had just stationed myself at an arm's length, but within whispering range of someone's baby, when before I even opened my mouth, I nearly jumped out of my skin. I didn't know if I'd activated something in the floor and inadvertently triggered the fire bell or if the parents had just arrived armed with a remote control to scare the daylight out of strangers and zap them away from their baby or what, but the moment it rang out, I recoiled and darted back to Marc's bedside.

It wasn't him. My line of vision leaped around the room looking for the source of the alarm. And then I heard another one. Shrieking. Echoing danger. Warning that someone had better come quick before the green line goes flat.

Monitors, hookups, ventilators, vital equipment. In any Intensive Care Unit, earnest, concentrated care is mandatory, obligatory. If not impelled by basic common sense, then the fundamental element of the profession and even rudimentary moral sensibility must be compelling enough to make one understand that there should be no allowance for not even one unguarded moment. In this respect, nurses are a lifeline.

Nobody came.

Frantic, I flew out of the room nearly running towards the nurses' station yelling.

"Help! Somebody get in here! The alarms! The alarms are going off!" Just as I got to the glass-walled partition of the nurses' station a few feet out into the hallway I stopped in my tracks. And then exploded. Clouds could have formed from the vapors I vented.

"What the hell is this? Don't you hear the alarms?"

A couple of them jumped out of their seats hastily snubbing out their cigarettes and quickly brushed past me.

I spun around after them.

"Have you lost your minds? How can you be up here smoking with these babies on respirators? How dare you? Where am I here? What kind of bullshit is this anyway?" I don't know how much of my enraged high-pitched English any of them understood. Nobody acknowledged a word I said. Didn't even look at me.

But I do know one thing: they got my message. And on the following evening in that intensive care unit, it was clear that all the givers of care working that previous night shift got the Professor's message as well. Helmut had called him at home and profusely expressed our shock, disappointment and absolute disbelief with regards to their behavior.

When they came on shift that evening, a couple of them were quite haughty. But they knew not to go too far. After my "Wahkoo" performance, (a daddyism), I'm sure they didn't know what to expect out of me next as it is so 'unGerman' to forsake one's mental poise and 'go off', or 'lose it', loudly, especially in public. I did not give a damn.

The truth of the matter is, there was no time for me to gauge a response. And I'll tell you this: looking at my baby and all those seriously ill babies, nearly round the clock, their tiny lives so very much in the balance, bound fast in tangles of intravenous lines, my fuse wasn't an inch long to begin with. Dunce in the first grade would understand that. I didn't care if they slighted me. I was self-exiled anyway. Even had this been a personal issue, I would not have fallen to their level as I don't believe that like can influence like, especially not in a negative manner.

Now, don't think this meant that I intended to ingratiate them. On the contrary. I had absolutely no feelings of apology or remorse for their getting reprimanded. The only thing I felt was an overwhelming expectation of them not to be remiss in the carrying out of their duties. I didn't have a problem pulling a Wahkoo and would do it again if necessary. It would just be best for everyone involved, for the nurses to administer to these babies, the purest and most rarified of creatures, like they meant it. Perform great deeds. Compatible with quality care.

To be honest, I didn't trust all of them to have a crisis of conscience so I kept my vigil as long as I could at Marc's side. I left him at one thirty that morning, lying on his back, his right cheek to the pillow.

When I arrived at six that morning, he hadn't been moved. A small portion of the curved fold that forms the rim of his outer right ear had in those hours developed an irritation.

I was ready to spit a bullet. Instead, I bit it. "Cultivate and try to maintain an inner peace," I kept telling myself. "Try. This too shall pass. His ear will heal. Stay focused on your goal: home."

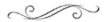

On the nineteenth of December we were released from the I.C.U. and sent back to the children's ward.

On Christmas Eve, the sepsis therapy was ended. That evening, Helmut and I sat side by side at his crib. Though we certainly didn't feel Christmas-carolly, our spirits were filled with songs of praise. We were beholden to God's Providence.

I found a blank piece of paper in my pocket calendar. Placed it next to Marc in the crib. I set the game up and showed Helmut how to play connect the dots. We played until all of the fields were closed, whereupon he wrote the words red and black in the boxes and taught me the principals of French roulette. And so was my second Christmas Eve in Germany.

And I gave glory on that holy night.

Two days later, Marc showed signs of an infection in his upper respiratory tract and water on his lungs.

At this point, I really began to wonder how I was going to slog my way through this. I'd been humbled. Brought to my knees. It made me call to mind all those times Mama said, "Tracie, you're only young once. You'd better enjoy your life." As if to say: There is something in this bigger than you. Be carefree as long as you can. You are young, a go-getter, enjoy it. But it's not yours to keep. In other words, you never know if or when life is gonna grab you.

Me? Hah! Life rolled on, one day into another and I thought I'd be young forever and problems, real problems were the stuff of novels and prime-time television. Now there was a blip on the screen of my life, the static filling me with an abject fear of the unknown, and the power that it wielded. Over me.

At once wilted and worn-out, nonetheless, my intrinsic determination was indestructible. I willed Marc to live and was convinced that I had to bring him to what I believed and would do it no matter what it took. The situation was bleak, but I just wouldn't have it, just wouldn't. In my heart, there was no denying the reality in my face, and I knew that this prizefight would be a severe test of stamina. That had been proven. And though it seemed as if God had said, "Okay, you want a baby? The most precious gift I can possibly bestow upon you? Are you worthy? Well, you're gonna have to work for it. Show me you are worthy."

In the end, I believed goodness would prevail. I just believed it. Even though, I still pondered over the fact that women had been giving birth since Eve, why did it have to be so extraordinary for me? I asked myself. And I thought about the world. And how my whole life I'd been spared the trials, tribulations, the twists, and tricks, the daily thorns in the flesh of the lives of many less fortunate than me. Considering all I'd seen, thankful for some of what I hadn't, I thought, "Well Tracie, honey, why not? Just why the hell not? Who do you really think you are?"

So I kept talking with God. I asked Him to help me develop all the emotional muscle I'd need to endure all the suffering He would keep my child free from.

I am confident that at our core lies our ability to reason. Reason gives our lives meaning, it infiltrates many, if not most of the choices we make and is superior to that part of us that lacks reason. It is greater, stronger, more productive, therefore it must be. In these dour circumstances, I knew I had every right to be afraid. And you know what? I was scared to death.

It was especially in the silence of the wee morning hours, when there was no twinkling in the black sky, that the demons would be on their worst behavior, clawing at my back, pulling me to my knees. And at the break of dawn, that moment when unconsciousness surfaced to consciousness, before I'd opened my eyes, that second my heart slipped out of gear remembering at once that something was wrong, it felt like a noose tightening around my neck as I tried to pull away. But I could not allow fear to coerce me into submission and leave me unable to function. I had to stay on my toes.

Within the very reaches of my soul, I reasoned that my fear had to be tempered with strength. I had no idea what I would yet have to face and had to be open to all possibilities as the unimaginable had already happened. But whatever it would be, if it was in the best interests of my child, I had to be ready for it. No matter what. I could not succumb to the angst. It would surely destabilize me. So I challenged fear to stimulate me, motivate and pull out the fight in me. Dared it to reveal the difference between the chickenshit and the chicken soup in my spirit. The result being that in a strange way, fear quickened my strength. This was the only way, I thought, that I would have the best vision to see our way out of this overwhelming realm of illness into one of wellness and promise. With God's blessing.

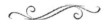

"You have to pat his back like I do," the nurse told me.

Imitating her motions, I leaned Marc's chest into my left hand and proceeded to lightly clap his back, my right hand arched, not flat. That was important that my hand was cupped. This had to be done several times a day, over the next several days, to loosen the phlegm from his lungs. On the sixth of January, the antibiotics were finished. Though he still had a pretty hefty cough going on, I felt that I could take just as good care of him at home and finally on the seventh of January we were free to go. Me, Helmut and our baby.

"*Sehr munter,*" the Professor remarked about our son upon our discharge. I smiled at Helmut's translation. He was very lively indeed I silently concurred.

Before we left, I was instructed how to administer his medicines and admonished to keep his environment as clean as I could. This of course meant sterilized in my book.

The grip of the plastic rattle was white with three multicolored spinning balls on its end. Of all the playthings in his room, I can't for the life of me remember why I picked up this particular toy. Guess I had to start somewhere. I'd figure out what to do with all the stuffed animals when I got that far. Everything had to be clean, free from bacteria and germs. So I filled a pot with water, sat it on top of the stove burner, brought the water to a rapid boil and dropped the rattle into the steaming bubbles. Just a minute or two should be enough, I thought. Was it ever. I removed it from the pot. It was no longer a rattle. It was now a glob that had melted into distortion.

You know, it's quite a coup when you reach the point where you can laugh at yourself. I mean really let 'er rip. The legs of the wooden chair grated against the stone floor as I pulled it out from underneath the kitchen table. I plopped down and laughed out loud. To the point of tears.

"Girlfriend, you're gonna have to learn when to hold 'em and when to fold 'em," I told myself.

"Well, I guess I should've just folded this one." And I cracked up again and wiped the tears from my eyes.

I needed that laugh.

CHAPTER FIFTEEN

Burgeoning Boy

Picture this: your baby boy, two and a half years old, perched upon your lap, torso reclined against your chest...You softly nuzzle the perfect crown of his head, the narrow nape of his neck, kiss your way around the curve of his silky jawline. He smells like baby powder and burgeoning boy. Transfixed by the a is for apple, b is for ball larger-than-life poster on the wall, he doesn't turn as he lifts his warm little hand to your face and sighs, "Ah, Mama," and the moment is a contented purr.

You are very keen for the Professor to finish jotting down his notes from the morning's checkup. Though swinging on tenterhooks, you nonetheless dare to feel victorious because the hammer hasn't fallen and much more than a sense of accomplishment, you feel like you've been moving mountains continuously fighting off the this virus and the that virus that have been afflicting your child, each time overcoming your own case of the frets because you are making progress: your child is alive, thriving and happy all over. You don't just feel good, damn it, you're batting a thousand!

And then you hear a shuffling of papers, the clink of a pen upon a table. The Professor speaks. He says, "He cannot survive. You should really think about having another baby."

You lift your eyes over your son's head. You stare the Professor in the face. Now, tell me. What do you say?

CHAPTER SIXTEEN

In a Tizzy

Three months later. No doubt I looked hideously unsettled. This was due in large part to wondering whether or not Helmut and I were doing the right thing. My lower limbs felt as though they were becoming unstuck from my torso, as if the muscles beneath the skin were melting reluctantly down cylinder extremities, clumping at my feet, making each step heavier than the one before, yet like good little soldiers, heel and toe continued to yield to circumstance and the carpeted gangway beneath my feet. Alternatively, simultaneously: I was downright slap-your-knee-kiss-your-grandpappy-giddy with glee!

With Marc fastened to my hip, I angled my way down the corridor. Contented, collected faces interrupted the catastrophic images blossoming in my mind.

"What if the Professor is right?" I kept asking myself.

All the preparations of the last weeks leading up to this very moment filled the far reaches of my mental heartland. The Professor's furrowed brow. "It's such a high risk," he said. "Not a good idea...perhaps a lack of oxygen...can't say for sure...you must ask yourself if this is really necessary...of course the authorities would have to be informed...if they'll allow it—"

"Would you do it?" I shot at him. He tilted his head and slightly shrugged his shoulders. His lips didn't bend. The look in his eyes told me to shelve the idea. I wanted to cry. I did cry.

And then I scrambled. Just the idea of having no option, of being shackled, seemed to squeeze my very essence into a claustrophobic vise-like grip. I made some calls. Based on the information I gathered, it was clear that this was not going to be easy. I surely would not get the Professor's cooperation. So I decided not to let the left hand know what the right hand was doing. I had to make this thing work.

After speaking with Dr. Tinschman, the world looked different: hope recovered. Part of our conversation centered on the fact that I needed a letter stating that despite Marc's heart defect, he was indeed in good health. "Not a problem," he told me.

This document was delivered to Dr. Sommer, the doctor in charge of the department of the company I thought could best accommodate us. He was extremely patient and kind and though we by no means locked horns, his demeanor indicated that he ran a shipshape department which was fine with me because as far as I was concerned, I'd done my homework: the letter he requested was in his hands. Thinking I had circuited the Professor's negative crosscurrent and that my mission was almost accomplished gave me such an adrenaline rush I nearly swooned.

A dream was about to come true and I was certain no thunderbolts were going to come hurling out of the sky striking me between the eyes. Yes! I thought, that oughta do it! And then? Dr. Sommer apologized for all my inconvenience, but he really did need to have the document signed by the Professor, the cardiologist. My engine reversed slap-bang! What? Didn't he understand I wasn't going to get a stamp of approval on a letter of this nature from the Professor? Why make it complicated? Did he need his own little personal guided tour of the state of no optimism? I was doing my damnedest to stay the hell away from there! Why wouldn't the letter he had in his hand suffice?

The necessity for Plan B had never occurred to me so I just tried to squirm my way out of this by feigning ignorance of German, German accented English and just basic common sense. To no avail. I was given a standardized form called a Medical Statement of the Diagnostician for the Professor to fill out. There was no getting around the issue. What could I do? All he could do was tell me no. And that would never suffice.

It looked as if the Professor had taken the document and slung the ink onto the page. His scribble and the paper appeared to be intentionally disconnected, the words looking as if they were in a hurry to go somewhere, like they were agitated, as if he'd reluctantly done the deed. With *Ach und Krach* as the Germans say.

"Marc may on and off need oxygen," he noted in answer to one of the questions. "Three to four liters per minute. His parents have expressed the wish for a medical attendant and will make the appropriate arrangements."

Ugh...Rewind, replay, rewind, replay. My brain must've looked like mincemeat. I didn't dare ask Helmut his opinion. No way. Not again. It was too late now anyhow. We'd been updownbackwards plus forwardsinsideout on this to the point that he finally believed (as I did deep in my heart, profoundly deep) that we were right-side up on this issue. Optimism is his virtue. He's adamant about not funneling energy into worrying until he has to. (I used to be like that, honestly.) And my response to that: okay, fine, great. But what if when you have to turns out to be too late?

"Tracie, then I would still deal with it then and not before!" I could hear him, his intonation a decimal higher than normal, just this side of pissed off. "Not even one minute before! So why should I worry me now? I am not *blöd*!"

"It doesn't have anything to do with being stupid, Helmut! I just won –"

"Stop it, Tracie! Just cut the mental masochism! You're losin' it, kiddo," I told myself. "Dr. Tinschman told you that you can't live in a glass house. And he also said that he didn't anticipate any problems. Life is for the living, so come on! Get a grip! Affirm everything good starting now! And lest you be confused, the Professor didn't swear on a stack of bibles, cross his heart, hope to die, sure as the Amen is in the church, guarantee in writing something would go wrong—"

"No he didn't, damn it! But he did say that if something happened it's not like a hospital would be right around the corner. And that's what scares the living daylight out of me. This goddamned if!"

"You don't have to be scared. You're not going to need a hospital. And in the unlikely event –"

Taptaptaptap...taptap! On my shoulder, startling me. I turned around and looked into his eyes.

"Frau Mayer, is everything alright?"

"Yes, Doctor Spatler. Thank you. Are you...are you okay?"

"Oh, yes, I'm fine, fine. Everything will be fine. Don't worry."

He patted my shoulder again and smiled a genuine smile. I smiled back. It was fake. I turned back around. Marc was getting restless, fidgety. I wished he would be still.

"...like I was saying," I continued telling myself, "if something happens, Dr. Spatler is here. I mean he's from the German Rescue Squad for Christ's sake. If you had any more of a security blanket, you'd probably smother."

"Yeah, but see, that's what I mean. Exactly the reason for my uneasiness. If everything is really going to be okay, then why is it even necessary that he's here?"

"What? You have to be kidding me, right? You know damn good and well why it's necessary; it's called Peace of Mind, Insurance, Whatever Gets You Through the Night, The Only Way This Whole Thing was Gonna

Happen – it was your choice. Be thankful that it all worked out. Be positive. No heebie-jeebies. No Professor phobia."

"I am thankful, it's just that –"

"I know, I know, I know, I know, I know. Marc is almost three years old now and we've come such a long, long way in that short time what with the colds and lung infections that dragged on for months and runny noses and fevers and vomitings and bronchitises and efforts to nip them all in their buds and taking it on the chin those times Dr. Tinschman gave the yellow light to the bugs belonging to the group of not-such-a-bad-guy viral infections, those ones conducive to building antibodies which every kid supposedly gets and worrying, worrying, worrying while we held them all under careful surveillance and then of course the almost weekly doctor visits and blood tests and the trips to the physical therapist...

"But hey! Now look! We made it! The antibiotics and cough medicines – they all worked! And after months of being rolled and pulled and encouraged, on a Monday afternoon you'll never forget, at two years, one month and twenty-six days this man-child stood up and took a first step and clapped his hands and yelled out "Bravo!" as he braved his next and you screamed and hollered until you were nearly hoarse and you know you'll always remember that time you overindulged his taste for chocolate pudding just so you could hear him say 'pud'n' till he eventually got the runs and—"

We were moving. "Oh my God, this is it. Breathe, girlfriend. Breathe. Think warm and fuzzy."

Marc's restlessness snapped me out of my thoughts. "Marc be still! Mommy means it, now, darn it!" I said, squishing him down between me and Helmut who at that very moment decided to reach over and affectionately squeeze my knee. I hate that.

"Calm, Tracie, calm. Cluster into yourself, feel the peace in this peaceful moment," I said to myself.

"Umhmm. Peace. Well...at least I won't be able to see this mass of stainless steel and hydraulics pitch and yaw and roll..."

"You're not exactly hang gliding here," I continued.

"You know, who would ever believe that I used to sit back, relax and just love this? And now I've got extra oxygen tanks packed away and medical assistance on standby from the German Rescue Squad and concerns about the physiological considerations imposed by pressurized cabins and these damned blotches are popping out on my face and my arms and I feel like a branding iron is poking me. I mean half the fun is supposed to be in the getting there! Isn't it? Will somebody please square this circle?"

"Are you finished?"

"I haven't even started."

"You might as well do what you've always done under these conditions."

"What's that?"

"Sit back and relax."

I finally quit talking to myself, sighed and briefly squeezed my eyes shut. The sound of takeoff swelled and soon we were soaring, soaring, soaring. Higher and higher until we reached our cruising altitude above bad weather and warnings, ribbons of air trailing the jetliner's logo.

Compass.

Control.

Cockpit.

This was it. After three years away from my native shore I was on my way back. I was actually, really and truly, finally taking Marc home!

I turned my fears over to the Autopilot. That one really in control, way up high.

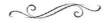

"Why won't this child stop fidgeting?" I asked myself.

Goodness gracious! He squiggled and wriggled and shifted nonstop from my lap to Helmut's, doddering and tottering along the armrests exchanging child's banter with the passengers behind, in front and to the sides of us who to my complete irritation kept initiating conversation with him in German, and seemed to get a kick out of watching him then talk to me in English, especially the flight attendants, particularly the one who brought him some flight souvenirs, one of which was a mini replica Lufthansa airplane and of course then it was "Wwwwwrrrrr, *gück mal mein Flugzeug Papa!*" and in the next breath it was "Wwwwwwrrrrr, look at my airplane, Mama!" and little arms laced the air but couldn't reach quite high enough which prompted little legs to aid in the ascent and it was as though he thoroughly, but thoroughly understood that this was his first trip on an airplane and that he was on his way to see his family and friends who lived far far away and there would be a mountain of love and kisses and toys and sweet, gooey Bonbons just for him and oh boy!

The adventure of it all and though it just seemed too good to be true, I was a wreck because I didn't know if all this activity was demanding too much oxygen of him which could possibly land us in a sea of trouble high in the sky, the very thought of which made me so nervous that Doctor Spatler had offered to give him a light sedative if that would reduce my tension.

"Is it necessary?" I asked him.

He laughed. "I really don't think so," he said.

"Good. Then just give it to me."

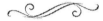

The plane landed without any lumps. We were all in a tizzy, and Mama and Daddy were just beside themselves.

We were standing, loaded down with grandchild, purse and carry-ons waiting to disembark. I couldn't believe it! I was finally here! With my child! With Helmut! And all of us in one piece! Suddenly, I saw an official-looking woman hastily making her way up the walkway through the throng of people crowding the aisle.

Her eyes glanced over Marc and then she looked to me. She spoke English. American English. Seattle English.

"Are you Mrs. Mayer?

What was this about? "Yes I am – why, what's the mat—"

She hurried on, "Is the baby alright?"

"Oh yes, he's fine! Great! We had no problems at all."

"Oh, well, that's wonderful," she said, "because we got a message that the child was ill and needed to be immediately expedited off the plane."

I didn't know who this woman was, how she knew us or anything about Marc. The flight was a breeze. Nobody called the Professor, the thought itself was ridiculous, and even if someone had – they would certainly not have had any troubling news – so what was that all about?

Daddy. He told the authorities on the ground just before we landed that there was a sick baby on board who had to immediately – that's read be the first – to disembark the plane. I was told that this was probably at about the same time Mama, overcome with emotion, anticipation and the hallelujah of it all let the lid slide off. She screamed.

"Theresa!" Grandma Ella, a lifelong family friend said.

Mama snapped her head in her direction and scowled. "You shut up!"

I don't think I've ever heard Mama say that like that and mean it to anyone – except Daddy. They just couldn't wait to see their grandson.

The first glimpse of the familiar faces of the bosom of my family electrified me. I didn't dare break my gaze; afraid heaven would disappear before my blurry eyes.

Unbelievable. The great divide was now reduced to just a few feet.

I handed Marc to Helmut and rushed into Daddy's opened arms.

"Hey sugar! There's my stuff!" He enfolded me in his arms, then stood back, looked at me, firmly wibble-wabbled my shoulders and pulled me close and hugged me ferociously again. I reached over and seized hold of Mama's neck and held on for dear life and my sisters clasped on and Auntie Christine and Gramma Ella were in there somewhere between all the squeezes and hugs and tears and shrieks of delight and "Oh my goodness, look at you! You look great! Girl, you do too! He's so big! How was Marc? How was the flight? Helmut, how you doin', son? Girl, how do you feel? Honey, you look wonderful. Did you have any problems? See? I told you everything would be alright! Just give it to the Man upstairs! How are you, honey? Look at my grandson! Ain't he fine – looks just like his granddaddy. Wipe those tears, you're home now! How was the flight? He's so cute! Giiiiirl, wait till we get home. Mama put on a pot of red beans and rice! Give me my grandchild. Just give him to me. Marc, honey, don't you want to come to Auntie Christine – your grandma don't want you..."

Marc became frightened at all the hoopla and Mama raised her arms and patted the air shushing us all into quiet. The moment was almost holy. Marc looked around at all the unfamiliar faces and shyly smiled. Daddy's nose looked kinda red, like how it did when he had a cold. I noticed his finger linger just a moment under the frame of his glasses as he adjusted them and his emotional center, but I knew what time it was with him. I was after all his Waterloo.

This was a memorable moment, underlined. It signified a salutation to "ain't no givin' up and no givin' out" and to "gettin' up and gettin' on it" and to guts and grit and survival, all the stuff Daddy's grandmama had taught him and what her forbearers had chiseled into her and how with single-minded intent, no matter how frayed his edges, he'd done his best to bequeath unto me bits and pieces of that inherited quilt, providing me with a pattern to weave my way amongst life's silk and bristle.

It was as well a tribute to Mama's optimism, her unwavering faith and belief in the power of prayer and in me to do my best in caring for her grandson and the countless times she comforted and consoled me and kissed it (albeit through the telephone receiver) all better. No wasted efforts by any means.

"I don't wanna hear that shit your grandma's talkin' 'bout," Daddy said reaching towards Marc. Oh well, so much for social graces.

"Come here to your granddaddy, boy."

He lifted Marc from Helmut's arms, leaving no room for disagreement and kissed him over and over again, grinning alternately at him and at each of us as he hammered his thumb back and forth into his chest. Marc chuckled.

"My grandson! Mine! A man-child!" he gushed. "Looks just like me. Tracie honey, you've finally done something right. You done good, girl. Made your daddy proud."

Horns blasted and a brass band played.

CHAPTER SEVENTEEN

Jumping Over Shadows

Buddha: "I do not fight with the world but the world fights with me."

Me: Everyone else cannot always be wrong.

"Hi everybody!" Marc said, waddling into the office, looking like sunshine waving his little hand at the group of men concentrated around the desk, instantly stifling the tongue-lashing Daddy was dishing out to them. The ranting and raving had gotten worse. Or maybe I'd just been away too long. Like a battering ram, he seemed to be hell-bent on destroying everything and everyone in his path, bless his soul. Spiked orange juice before noon only exacerbated his discontent.

I don't know if he feared that hurricane within, or if he just couldn't stop it, but what I do know is that in a heartbeat, this can all be gone. So why whittle away at the gem when by its very nature it is rough around the edges? Why not smooth away the unnecessary ruggedness and raggedness within the realms of possibility and find the solid goodness? And then, rest satisfied, blessed with contentment in knowing that you have all one could ask for. Especially at fifty-three years old.

Mama, trailing her grandson, entered the office just as the last man out had quietly shut the door behind him. Rolling her eyes at Daddy she swept Marc up from his lap, said, "Come to your grandma, Sugar Lump," and carried him to the kitchen for breakfast. Good thing Marc was her armor because she would've more than likely incurred Daddy's wrath for 'looking at him the wrong way' and I don't necessarily mean wrathful words. I had settled myself on one of the vacated hot seats. This of course opened the door.

"They are some stupid assholes!" Daddy said. Reflexively, I ducked back, unsure if the pen he had struck hard onto the desk would spring back my direction. "Tell 'em the same goddamn thing over and over again and they still don't get it! They just can't think! I'm so sick of holdin' everybody's hand I could scream!"

"Calm down, Daddy."

"Oh calm down my ass! I—"

"You know, you're gonna have to lower your voice – your grandson is not used to all this screaming and foul language. I don't want him to be afraid of you."

"Oh bullshit! That's a man-child. But speaking of my grandson, I think it's a shame that you're raising him so far away from me..."

"Daddy –"

"...and your mama and your sisters."

"Daddy—"

"You need to move back home and—"

"DADDY! What needs to happen is that you stop! Just stop. And listen to yourself. Take a moment to reflect. Lay down your artillery. Hear yourself when you address people or shall we more accurately say, jump down their throats. You can't keep going around berating and belittling everybody and the way you talk to Mama and the girls is just deplorable! Nobody wants to be treated like that. You wouldn't like it. What's wrong with you?"

"Listen honey," he said and cleared his throat. "I am still the good feeder around here – ain't nothin' changed – and as long as everybody is up underneath my umbrella – he, she, mutt, cat – whatever – they will do as I say do."

"Oh, Daddy, pleeease. This rhetoric is so antiquated."

"You don't understand, sugar! All of 'em are dummies – I can't get a goddamn thing done for havin' all this dead weight around me..."

"You know, you're beginning to sound foolish and you are not a stupid man. It would behoove you to banish the bullshit, Daddy. I'm serious. Before it's too late."

"Okay, I promise I'm'll behoove and reflect. I just need you to come back home and help me run the business. You don't have no business bein' in Germany anyway. You're a big girl, a fine girl, and you've proved your point so you need to just go on back over there, pack your bags and bring your ass back home."

"There was no point to prove and further—"

"Well, you proved it anyway so I want you to just get on the plane, get your stuff together and get back over here. You can bring the dog. You gotta dog, don't you?"

I chuckled and shook my head. Daddy, Daddy, Daddy...They threw away the mold when he escaped the hatch.

So there we were. Not exactly uncomfortable, it was more of an unfamiliar quiet that weighed in around us as we sat staring at one another, the film of our lives, the sum and substance, rolling reel to reel between us.

"Your mama can take care of the baby," he finally said.

Mama would surely have taken care of Marc, but that was not the only issue. What, for example, about Helmut and his business and our life? I couldn't expect him to unhitch his wagon from his star and pack up and move to Seattle just 'because Daddy said to'. And I had absolutely no intention of subjecting him to the Good Feeder's "my way or take the highway" mentality. That would have been the quickest way to end my marriage and didn't even come into question.

I slumped back in my chair weary with sorry for my father, for mom, the girls, for me, and for Marc and the milestones that Helmut and I could only interpret for them. Shitty situation. It really tore my heart out, but what could I do? Germany really was east of the sun and west of the moon from here and as much as I wanted to, I could not straddle the ocean. And even if I could have worked a wonder, it would have been too late. Decisions had been made. Unbudgeable decisions. Things would never be the same again. Sometimes when we have the *nase voll*, as the Germans say, or 'have had it up to here', as Mama said, that happens.

Unbeknownst to Daddy, she was about to make her move and my sisters, who for all practical purposes were living on their own anyway, would be joining forces with her.

Sadly, and so misfittingly, in the not too distant future, strangers would lay claim to these walls and at Christmas time they would snip bits of the spiny green leaves and red berries away from the knoll of holly shrubs; and when the yellow fleshy pears hung just right from the tree that pillared uncultivated near the office door, someone's feet would begin to climb her and on a perfect summer morning, somebody else would happen to glance down at the pool from the kitchen window, do a double take, and fly out the front door, dash around the porch, stop, look down and marvel at the mottled brown mama duck floating contentedly about the blue waters of the pool, her tribe of ducklings paddling quickly behind her – but for now, this was still my home.

I brought my child here so he could breathe the air I'd breathed, see the lakes and magnificent mountains I'd seen and meet the many people I knew and loved. And play with Sheba, the family dog. It didn't matter that he was too young to understand the significance of it all or that nothing more than mere snapshots would have the power to perpetually evoke places and voices from the past. For us all. Especially me.

Neither Marc, nor Helmut nor I ever saw my father alive again.

So, yes, Professor, to answer your question, this trip was necessary. Very necessary. In more ways than one. Or two or a million.

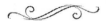

Since the day of his prognosis, I very much looked forward to having Marc examined by a doctor stateside. Dr. French, Professor of Pediatrics, had a disposition as sunny as that August day Marc and Mama and I visited.

The results of the physical exam concluded that "at two years-nine months Marc was growing at a reasonable level. The echocardiography demonstrated a functional two- chambered heart...that has been well supported with his shunts. The cutaneous oxygen saturation today was eighty-four percent...Marc certainly has complex cyanotic heart disease," he further noted in his report.

"To date, he has made reasonable progress with a pretty standard approach through his pulmonary atresia problem. The next steps in terms of some kind of modified Fontan or perhaps ultimately even consideration of some kind of transplant technology will be an extremely difficult one. Hopefully, the techniques and understanding of the Fontan type operation will continue to develop, and perhaps at the time Marc requires a more definitive procedure, a better answer will be available."

Hopefully is the key word here; it was my foothold as I carried my son out of the Seattle Children's Hospital and Medical Center, Mama's arm draped around my shoulder.

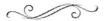

And then, before I knew it, it was time to go back to Germany. Time to go...home. And on that day, feeling certain and uncertain, so full of yes, no, and I don't know, it hit me. I realized that having a finger immersed in the flavorful pie of life requires personal evolution, and sometimes revolution, whether we like it or not, for it is not an easy task to understand our needs and wants and choices and why we need and want and choose them and wracking our brains out trying to justify it all. And no matter if we're flying towards the opposite side of the world, getting a divorce or just learning to adjust to a different situation, the sheer force of the circumstance thankfully helps us to jump over our own shadows.

Everyone would find his way, I decided. For even in a dim light, life does indeed go on.

CHAPTER EIGHTEEN

Learn By Doing

Helmut's and my long-distance courtship lasted a little over a year. During that time, I visited Germany twice, each time for two weeks and he came to America four times, each time staying several weeks. In between these visits, we spoke daily on the telephone.

In May of 1984 we got married in Seattle. A week before our wedding we found out that I was three months pregnant and we were ecstatic. We headed to Germany a week after our wedding and although leaving my family was extremely difficult and saddened me, I felt nonetheless elated: I was a wife and soon would be a mother!

When I permanently arrived in Germany, I knew really next to nothing about the language or the culture. The only thing I was certain of, was that Helmut and I were deeply, passionately in love and couldn't wait for our child to be born.

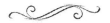

A couple days after we got unpacked and began to get settled in our home, I remember thinking: You're gonna have to learn how to cook. But before this fait accompli, I had to figure out what it was I intended to cook. To that end, Helmut took me to a massive grocery store; everything from beef to portraits of the Balkan Sea congregated under one roof. He meant well.

"So sweetie," he said. "Here's the milk. See? And over there is the bread, all different kinds and look, on that side over there is the fresh fruit and *Gemüse* (vegetables). See?"

"*Gemüse*," I repeated. "Spell it, please."

"G-e-m-ü-s-e, " he said.

"Um-hmm," I said. One word, hard g, I thought.

"And down this aisle are *Zeitschriftungen* and magazines..." His voice trailed off as he picked up a daily newspaper, turned to the sports section and became engrossed with the headlines. Pirouetting clockwise, anti-clockwise and clockwise again, certain an onset of stereoscopic vision would pinpoint something, anything to make me shout out, "Yeah! I recognize that!" I was nearly dizzy by the time I realized it was a no-go and then, suddenly, my enquiring mind posed the following fair question: Where are the feminine hygiene products?

He stole a glance at his watch, started getting antsy. It wasn't that his store, Maytex, was such a big floor-covering store; he was just uncomfortable leaving the only salesman he had, other than himself, alone there for any real length of time. Neither did he pine over grocery shopping.

Well, as far as I was concerned, we could hurry up and jump back in the car because this hypermarket destroyed all my notions of romantic sentiment. I'd go later by myself, somewhere a bit cozier, closer to our apartment, where the neighbors shopped. Hopefully someplace where I could within a few days establish a rapport with the employees so that with their help, my shopping dilemmas would quickly develop into deliberate choices. Until then, I would have to slowly get a feel for things.

Let me put it this way: fruits were easy. An apple is an apple all over the world. Thank goodness. Just into the beginning stages of my pregnancy, I didn't have to be concerned with buying baby food and all that. No doubt the hospital or my gynecologist would fill me in on that later. Right now, experiencing my first attempt at solo grocery shopping, I needed to know what the hell packaged salt looked like.

My eyes poured over the stocked shelves as I inched forward and backwards along each section of the secret food and nonfood stuffs, picking up this box and that bag, squeezing, shaking, sniffing, scrutinizing. Carefully.

"Well girlie. You can stand here and chew the cud over these packages till the very last cow comes home," I said. "But you and I both know the only way to find out what's inside these packages –"

I turned around to see if anyone was behind me.

"...is to take a little peek inside."

Blue box. White diamond on the front, red trim bordered the top, snow-capped mountain range skirted underneath...I peeled the corner away, tilted a smidgeon of its contents into my hand, and took it to my mouth. SALT! Pierced a hole in a bag. SUGAR! When I wasn't carefully tearing open corners and stabbing holes in the tops of packages and stealthily placing them back on the shelves, pictures on the labels determined if this can or that jar would make it into my basket.

So Operation Figure It All Out Because You were Excited about the Expedition and Forgot the Dictionary at Home went on like this until my little shopping cart contained a few basics, as well as some fixings for dinner, but not too much to load me down for the ten-minute walk back to the apartment. Tomorrow would be a new day. I'd get the hang of this – despite the fact that the cooking directions on the bag of frozen *Pommes Frites* (french fries) were only in German, Czechoslovakian, Polish, Spanish and Italian.

There was no one waiting in line at the checkout counter. It was twenty minutes past noon, and not knowing if it was still okay to say *"Guten Morgen"* (good morning) or if *"Guten Tag"* (good day) was more suitable at this time of day, and not trusting myself to voice either correctly, I thought the best thing to do was to greet the cashier with a smile. She didn't respond. "Maybe she's having a bad day," I thought. "We all do now and then. Don't take it personally."

"Maybe she saw you opening a package," I said to myself.

"Yeah well, maybe she didn't," I answered.

"Hmmm…"

Ignoring myself, I sat the basket on the counter and waited. Out of the corner of my eye, I detected other customers queuing up behind me so I plopped my purse down and started digging in a race against time through everything inside for my wallet. I guesstimated that all my purchases would just about fill a bag, so with wallet in hand, I was prepared to pay, sling my purse strap over my shoulder, throw my wallet on top of the bagged groceries, scoop the bag up, smile good-bye, be out of everybody's way and out of there.

I waited. The cashier waited. The people in line waited. The cashier looked at me. I smiled. She didn't. Beads of sweat began to break out on my forehead. Not having a clue as to why she sat there immobilized, I ever so slightly nudged the metal basket carrying my goods closer to her, placed my wallet down on the counter in front of my stomach, and with raised eyebrows, opened palms and a sheepish shrug, I smiled again and nodded foolishly trying to convey: "That's it. That's all for today. You can ring 'er up now. Tee-hee." Even though her dour face said it all, she nonetheless mumbled something at me. I figured she'd understand Please before she would Excuse me so that's what I said.

"Please?" I asked, my eyes wide and begging with question, my moral sensibilities willing to wager ALL my money that she would take my hand and guide me around this little impasse and not let me topple over into that lonely chasm of absolute utter embarrassment in front of the other customers. There were only two cash registers in this store. The other started suddenly ringing. Glancing up, I'd found my savior. The shopper was removing her items from her basket and placing them on the counter. Those items were being rung up. Aha! Monkey see, monkey do. Quickly.

A wave of relief washed over me as I watched my cashier's fingers deftly tip the price of each of my items onto the keys of the *Kasse*, then push the item itself to the side. But before I even had a chance to enjoy my crumb of comfort, she had reached a total, all my purchases were piled in one heap at the end of the counter and I was standing there trying to go with the flow, doing my best not to appear uncouth as I ignored her muffled gobbledygook and directed my attention beyond the expectant look on her face to the neon numbers glowing on the cash register because not only could I not read, I could not count! Not verbally! Tallying the currency was no problem. But *neun und vierzig acht und siebzig*??? Sounds like a trick, doesn't it? She might as well have said "Abracadabra."

Well, this *neun* (nine) *und vierzig* (forty), *acht* (eight) *und siebzig* (seventy) was the amount of my bill. Now, why go through the horrors of reversing the numbers when it's just plain old forty-nine (German Marks at that time) and seventy-eight (cents)? I mean what was up with that? So all this was going on while I fumbled about with the money in my wallet wondering if she would be nicer to me or at least be pleasant if I gave her the exact change down to the *Pfennig* (penny) while at the same time reprimanding myself because I was just too lame-brained to get it that if she hadn't smiled yet, it was unlikely that she planned to, especially when her customers waiting behind me began to "tsk" and sigh audibly as they shifted their weight from one leg to the other and on top of all this, there was nary hide nor tail of a bag boy in sight. Dropping the change from a fifty Deutsch Mark bill into my hand, she asked me something. Tossing the coins harum-scarum into my purse, I looked at her and thought, "Good grief, lady. I mean, where do we go from here?"

She reached down beneath her counter and pulled up a grocery bag and waved it at me. Would I like a grocery bag? Yes! Yes! Of course! I gave her the peace sign and got two. I'd seen the other shopper who saved my situation bag her groceries, so I hurriedly doubled the bags, tossed in the goods from the day's venture and scurried like the dickens out of there.

CHAPTER NINETEEN

P is for...

I'd come a long way since that time several years ago when I first arrived in Cologne, yet I was still very much preoccupied with getting into the swing of living in one of Germany's oldest cities. My top priority of course: the well-being of my family. Helmut and I had our ups and downs, but despite all the out of the ordinary obstacles we dealt with, or maybe because of them, for many years, we remained in sync.

By this time, my grocery shopping was down pat as to what I bought where. Meat, for example, came from the *Metzgerei*, (butcher) with the red and white awning hanging over its front door around the corner from our house. Wednesday and Saturday mornings would find me contentedly treading home from the local neighborhood farmer's market toting bags of fresh fruits, veggies, eggs and a bunch or two of colorful blossoms. A scrumptious assortment of perhaps thirty to forty varieties of bread, (at times still too warm to slice), *Brötchen*, bigger-than-your-hand-sized pretzels and an array of "um, um, ummm!" pastries could be bought at any *Bäckerei*, a myriad of which fingerprinted the cityscape. General household incidentals I picked up here and there, depending on the prices.

I was very particular about our heart-healthy meals and thankful that I had the time to devote the care towards preparing them, especially Marc's diet during this time; iron was the particular issue here: too much in his little system could induce excess red blood cells to cultivate, resulting in a thickening of his blood. The hemoglobin test, that indicator of the blood's ability to carry oxygen throughout the body, always held the answer. A value over eighteen or nineteen pushed the limit. Twenty was considered too high.

Even if the doctors said it wouldn't make a difference, and though Marc was still not a voracious eater, it took me all of a nanosecond to decide that whether he ate a lot or a little was irrelevant, he was still what he ate, so the only logical step in my mind was to control how often and how much iron-rich foods he consumed. Couldn't hurt. Couldn't be too careful.

During this time, hemoglobin checkups were carried out by Dr. Tinschman, Marc's pediatrician, in his office every four to eight weeks. A prick of a predominate vein, the seeping of rich ruby red fluid inside the vacant walls of a colorless vial, a Band-Aid, and then the agonizing wait until the following day for the results. Inhale, exhale, hemoglobin check to hemoglobin check.

So busy concentrating on living, focusing primarily on keeping Marc healthy, the forefront of my consciousness was not mindful to the fact that the moment was slowly creeping up on me when I would have to look into the pure soul of his child eyes and be forced to tell him about his cardiovascular disease. I mean, of course I knew the day would eventually come – I just...sort of set it on the back burner and...and left it there to quietly simmer.

I guess it's also safe to say that I didn't want to deal with it. The Cowardly Lioness: at times Herculean she thinks she is, however, Hercules she is not. If the truth be told, I would have honest to God preferred eating shit with the buzzards. How this thing preyed on my mind! He was just a child for Christ's sake! The last thing I wanted or needed was to create tension in a little mind where up till now none existed, yet I knew he had to be told. Good grief! So there I was going round and round completely at a loss as to what I should say and how I should say it, feeling damned if I did and damned if I didn't and nobody could find the key to open the door to my airtight quandary...and the mental flagellation would not let up.

Helmut would be unblenching, of course. I needed no reassurance there, but this wasn't really his domain. By the time he twisted the key in the lock, activated the alarm and secured the store premises until the next working day and drove the five or so minutes home, Marc would be freshly bathed, lotioned, powdered, fed, medicined and ready for Papa to play *Patchi Patchi Futili*. I knew it would be up to me to put on the kid gloves and point out the rainbow over this whole thing. I swear it can seem like you're doing all you can with all your might and there are still times when the parenting profession can grind you down, trample on you and just drain you for all you are worth.

I brooded over 'this could be a traumatic event' persistently and came to the conclusion that how this information was conveyed to him could be a pivotal point in Marc's young life: it could in fact break his spiritual and/or emotional steadiness and very well determine whether he would sink or swim through life. Sinking would surely not work, so that meant these waters had to be tread carefully. Marc would have to get used to the situation because he was going to have to live with himself. And more importantly, like himself. For life. I summed it up this way: Learning early on to accept and like himself would lead to a wholesome mental well-being, and create a sense of ease, rather than dis-ease.

The tie between that rhythmically contracting fist-sized muscle tissue pumping blood through our bodies and our emotions cannot be cut loose. Just consider how independent of our conscious control, it beats faster when we are excited or when we detect fear or danger or a love interest. Another dimension to ponder is that of the ancient Greeks who believed that the heart is the seat of intelligence. Without question, it is indeed our chief thing; the rhythm of life.

A steady cadence, one free of the tremors and quakes that result from mulling about in mental squalor, would be the foundation of overall good general health for my son. And I was sure Marc had the basics because he was such a happy as a habit, carefree kind of kid.

So I could not afford to mess this up. Wisdom after the event would not help me, so I prayed. Good Lord, how I prayed. Over the years I'd been putting it through some serious wear and tear, but it was the only pillar I had to cling to, so I embraced it tightly as I begged for the strength to find a real good hiding place for my anxieties and for the wisdom to gently deliver this disclosure to our son in bite-sized chunks so that he could get just enough of the overview, but not so much that it set off an alarm in his preschool imagination that dredged up from his psyche a long crooked hairy bloody finger with prickly things sticking out all over it that grew even longer when he cried and pointed out the wrong shoe for the wrong foot and to monsters under his bed; nor should it trigger excuses to morph molehills into mountains, and I especially prayed that it wouldn't snuff out that golden tone that tinkled in his laughter.

Helmut and I had been raising Marc like we would any child. There was a time when he was young, that I was accused of packing him in cotton – but that's just not true. I see it otherwise: It's a 'p' word alright – but it is p as in protection, which I will go into in a minute. Nonetheless, he was disciplined, well-mannered and knew his limits. You could take him anywhere and you'd never know he was in the room. Which reminds me of a scene Helmut and I witnessed at the Clinic in Düsseldorf at the time of Marc's first operation...

Sitting in a room off the hallway of the Children's Ward when a young boy and his mother entered and settled themselves across from us, Helmut and I reflexively glanced up at them; our gazes then fell back to our clasped hands on my lap.

And then back to them. The child, clad in a hospital gown, was about five or six years old. He apparently must've chosen the chair with the sharp ends of porcupine quills on the seat. A rumble developed between him and his mother just as they sat down. The poor woman whispered while he hissed. She tried to wrap her arm around him and he jostled away, opened the mouth on his contorted little face and started yelling at her. Viciously. How could one so little foster such mammoth anger? She patiently cooed, lovingly tried to stroke his hair and pat his arms. He responded by slapping her hand and swatting at her like she was just too many flies. Helmut and I just stared.

This little drama escalated to the point that a nurse picked up the commotion from out in the hallway somewhere and came in to try to help the mother quiet this child. Then all of a sudden he screamed. The only part of this litany I understood or even paid any attention to were the first two words. I couldn't get any further, even if I had understood what all his racket was about. Helmut couldn't figure out if he was letting loose on the mom or the nurse. *"Du Schwein!"* he screamed. (You pig!). *"Du Schwein, Du Schwein!"*

The only thing I remember thinking was Oh, hell no!

Marc was not a bed-wetting, whining, afraid of the dark, nightmare having kind of kid. And he never, ever complained before or after a doctor visit. Needle or not. Not ever. I don't understand it, but I'll always thank him for that. How many lucky stars did I count, so very grateful that he didn't make me feel even more like dying than I did by causing a scene in preparation for a doctor visit.

And because the onslaught of infections didn't lighten up, there were weeks when it seemed that we spent more time at the doctor's office than we did at home. If he had developed a real anxiety and snotted and squirmed and carried on I don't know how I would have been able to bear it. It was horrible enough to squeeze him tight and tell him not to look while I forced myself to watch a needle pierce and penetrate his skin.

Once into toddlerhood, the sharp pain of these pricks no longer made him cry, and like always, his courage encouraged me. Courage, how absolutely fitting its etymological meaning: heart. And on top of all this, he was always cheerful. This was Helmut's and my, as the Germans say, 'Glück im Unglück'. Fortune in misfortune.

I can't say how he physically felt at this time. I would dare to guess that because he knew no other way to feel and in light of the fact that he never mentioned it, when he ran out of breath and had to take a *Pause*, that he considered this, well, inconsiderable. When no longer winded, he would carry on with whatever it was that he was doing.

Maybe he was too young to fathom otherwise. Perhaps his spirit soared on the wings of angels high above his compromised circumstance – I really don't know, but it was as if Marc dealt with the situation on another level and I didn't care – no matter right or wrong, I consciously did all I could to protect that. Alas, that 'p' word.

Though he suffered not even a little bit from stranger anxiety, there were no children his age on our block and quite honestly, I didn't go out of my way to expose him to other kids. I'll explain. First of all, there was the infectious bacteria thing. This was a serious problem. So serious that Dr. Tinschman instructed me to bring him in whenever I deemed necessary – without appointment – as long as it was no later than eight in the morning, so that we could get in and out before the other children crossed the threshold with their infectious ailments. (Now that I think back, I wonder why it didn't enter my mind to ask if the germs from the day before could survive through the night. I guess that's what years of worry will do to you: take your mustard seed sized brain and render you an anxiety suffering, excessively preoccupied candidate for a professional diagnosis and treatment plan.)

And secondly, because at four years, Marc was a delicate child who tired not long after the onset of any physical activity, I wanted to spare his feelings and the "why can't I and why can they?" questions of it all. And spare myself the agony of his eyes searching mine for an answer.

But, just because I didn't go out of my way in search of playmates doesn't mean that I deprived him totally of contact with little people.

Take a look for example at this entry from my calendar on Friday, August 5, 1988: call lady for Marc to play, tel.79277. This lady was a mom Marc and I met at our first visit to the neighborhood playground. It wasn't a sign of rudeness that I didn't register her name at our introduction, it's just that on that premier visit, my undivided attention shadowed Marc uninterruptedly. Though he immediately acclimated himself to play, it took my on the alert for any mishaps eagle eye a while to register that. Once assured he was happily occupied, my eyes and ears quickly surveyed the elements: a handful of squealing kids scattered about, a four-cornered sandbox splayed out beneath a larger-than-life jungle gym whose blue metal loops arched high in the air and were crisscrossed by orange and red bars, just perfect for daredevils, a pair of wooden orange and yellow squeaky teeter-totters and four thick, coarse, free swinging braided ropes that hung suspended from a plank high as a giraffe's head off the ground, and finally, my eyes squinted into vision the total number of stairs it took to get to the top of the slide.

I didn't fret that I would sound like an idiot that first time I called lady and couldn't remember her name because the Germans usually answer the telephone with their last names rather than with hello anyway. And the mere fact that I actually stuffed her telephone number (albeit inattentively) into my purse was a sign of good intention.

Our little outings to the playground led to visiting a few playgroups, but after a while, 'this appointment came up' and then 'that one was sick' and then of course, "*Nein, Heute nicht – ich habe keine Zeit.*" ("No, not today – I don't have time.") popped up to the point that the group eventually abandoned itself.

We hobnobbed when the time allowed with Hilda, the lady we'd met at our first visit to the playground, and her two young boys. Though she couldn't speak English, she deciphered my staccato German very well, and was very easy, very likable. Though her two boys could at times be rambunctious, they were nice kids and played well with Marc.

Several months after we'd met, Hilda and her family moved to another part of the city and though she or I would occasionally pack up the kids for the drive along the Autobahn to visit each other, that too petered out. The loner in me could deal with that, but it was too bad that Marc had lost a couple of familiar playmates.

Though my linguistic form improved steadily, it still remained a stumbling block, if not at times an outright irritation for me. I hadn't met many moms who could converse fluidly or even thickly for that matter in my mother tongue, and few who didn't stare at my nails or what I was wearing when they spoke to me, or who weren't so Boom! in my face direct about Marc:

"Wieso atmet er so schwer?" they'd want to know. ("Why does he breathe so heavy?")

To satisfy the curiosity of these acquaintances, I would lightly graze the edge of our situation by replying, *"Mein Sohn hat einen Herzfehler."* ("My son has a heart defect.") Whereupon they'd pull out the shovel:

"My good gracious! What exactly is the problem, a hole in his heart? Will he need another operation? He's had two already?! What kind of operations were they? Will he need another? How long do the doctors say he can live?"

How long can he live? How people can actually give voice to shameless delving and probing into the sensitive affairs of another and not bat an eyelid is beyond me. It's on the same level as gawking at someone different, less fortunate or other than we are – the foolish act itself defines the person behaving in this manner. What I want to know is: Who issued the permission slips allowing boorishness?

Unfortunately, my experience has been that if allowed, this kind of insensitive ignorance can go on and on. Did I consider it to be prying? Definitely. Well meaning? I don't know. In any event, the result of being exposed to such callousness, immediately unplugged the connection for a possible friendship as far as I was concerned. In a nutshell, I had no interest to sip coffee over cake, seeking for the sake of my child a friendship that sapped my energy, and made me feel like my son and I were the variants, constantly observed and where some shallow-minded female's curious needling would leave me wondering what the next spine chiller out of her mouth would be.

Motherhood does indeed share certain universal truths, but the function itself of giving birth does not make one privy to an all-exclusive club. We all have our shortcomings, but a woman having the tender feelings of a scrub brush fell way below the mark.

Needless to say, the offspring of these women were not considered playmates for Marc. Our children, these little extensions of ourselves, learn what we teach them. If a mother inclined toward rudeness, well, sometimes the apple doesn't fall too far from the tree. I didn't dare leave it to chance that her youngster would know to behave any better than his primary example. We all of course are familiar with how cruel children can be; take a moment and remember back...

Swelling the ranks of more kid stuff to do with kids, playdates did occasion, like with the Benz boys, the sons of family friends Gerd and Sabine, and a select other few children I allowed Marc to meet with preferably at our house for temperate play. No roughhousing was the rule. That was understood. And these kids just wanted to play for playing's sake; no notice was given to or comment was made on the state of Marc's health.

It was indeed fulfilling just to be in the moment, interacting with Marc from that part of me that's bred in my bone with no unnecessary stresses. I thrilled in watching him thrive. Everyday presented something new or something improved, something to show Papa when he got home from work. Nothing, not one thing was taken for granted. Each day proved to be a more huggable humdinger than the one before.

The Professor was continuously updated on Marc's progress at our checkups every six to twelve months, or by telephone when I'd place an enquiry call about something in between. When one considered our humble beginnings at the jump street, I'd say that a little better than four years on down the road, we'd been making great big huge strides!

Despite this, when Helmut spontaneously reached out for me from a sound sleep, as he was wont to do, with more and more frequency he would find that the strong-arm tactics of insomnia had left a dead of night void beneath my sweaty sheets and rumpled blankets.

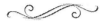

At a checkup in January of 1989, justifiably proud, Helmut and I reeled off to the Professor all about our well-adjusted kid who grew sturdier by the minute, enjoyed the company of others, but also contentedly entertained himself, imaginatively played in his room with his toys and sang softly as he assembled picture puzzles advanced for his age.

The Professor responded in typical fashion, reiterating his forecast that we shouldn't expect Marc to be physically active, that sometimes these children are intelligent because they have no choice but to sit quietly and read or think or whatever. (I wondered: How does he know this when I distinctly remember him telling me when Marc was born that these babies usually die? He must've meant the ones that fell outside the usual category or perhaps this was an assessment based upon later enquiry or research or both or...I don't know.) The consequence being he continued, that he probably would get fat and in all likelihood probably be short and perhaps develop clubbed fingers and toes, spin-offs of his illness.

"Tracie, deal with this real quick, while he's got the stethoscope in his ears. Put it into perspective and get over the hump so you can focus on the rest of this exam," I told myself.

"Gosh, no kidding. I'd better pull myself up by my bootstraps right now," I thought. "So, here's my take on all this: I don't give a damn about Marc running around playing sports anyhow and there are a whole lot of kids in the world who don't give a hoot about athletics either, so he won't necessarily be singled out from that standpoint and besides, only a select few bounce and bang balls against their heads and actually get paid anyway, God forbid they break a leg, so this news really does not affect me – I have absolutely no intention of veering away from the decision I came to before he had even been tucked inside my womb and that is to concentrate on developing his mind.

And that's final. And I know Helmut's with me on this. Now, between Marc's naturally thin physique and my low-fat kitchen, I don't anticipate him having a weight problem. And as for the long and the short of it? Helmut doesn't come from tall people, but I do. And we'll just pray that his fingers and toes don't change. So. Enough about that for the time being. Put it away till later."

I couldn't deal with what 'could probably' happen right now. Testing my margin of endurance recently was the fact that I couldn't tell if Marc was looking puffy and maybe more cyanotic under the eyes and under his fingernails. At times, his lips. Helmut did his best not to let his own butterflies flutter. I tried not to see what I wasn't sure I saw. See...? Saw...? See...saw...see, saw, seesaw, seesaw . . .

I wasn't alone. At the past couple checkups, the Professor's opinion also wavered. That's why he'd asked me to come to this appointment with unpainted fingernails. If both Marc's parents had been German, the cyanosis would be clearly visible and the doctors surely would have confirmed his heart ailment sooner if not immediately after his birth.

The Professor took my hand in his and studied the bed of my fingernails. Looked at Marc's. Reached for my other hand, Marc's. Pursed his lips, shrugged his shoulders. Removing the polish hadn't steered him any closer towards the truth; he still couldn't tell if Marc's coloring was due to cyanosis or because he was half black.

There was something else: Marc's breathing. It seemed to have become more labored, so much that sometimes, by the time he slowed to stillness, he would be gasping. I attributed this to the high heat of summer and/or the labors of an infection. This year alone he had been on antibiotics three times for pneumonia, the last bout ending just a couple of weeks ago. Even today the Professor detected the stray whispers of bronchitis during the aural examination. Runny noses. Ear infections. Colds. Lung infections. As often as you like.

Fortunately, relief came in the form of good news that day: The results of the exam showed his oxygen level hovered between 80 and 85 percent, the hemoglobin level at 16.5 percent, nothing negative had developed, therefore no need to consider an alteration of our present course. The Professor, pleased with Marc's psychomotor development, instructed me to continue with his medication, regular hemoglobin checkups and an endocarditic prophylactic therapy if the need arose, which meant he should take an antibiotic if he had any kind of medical procedure involving the risk of a bacterial infection getting in his bloodstream; dental surgery for example. He could not explain from a cardiological point of view the dyspnea, so as long as his shortness of breath had nothing to do with an ailment of his heart, that was genuinely fine, fine, fine by me. It was just something we would live with.

The examination was over. The Professor had momentarily left the room. We three hugged tightly and giggled real quickly before he came back. We were always doing that.

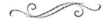

As the days went by, Marc and I were never short on supply of things to do. Mama kept United Parcel Post in business with the boxes and boxes of books and talking toys, stuffed animals and games she sent. I bought alphabet books and learning activity toys in German. 'The Cat in the Hat' and *'Die Biene Maja'* got equal play in our house.

And we played and brought to life the tales we spun and the stories we read, and over and over again I vividly told him the narrative of the little engine that chugged and toiled and tugged along the railroad track puffing "I-think-I-can-I-think-I-can-I-think-I-can" until she finally reached the top of the mountain and puffed out, "I thought I could! I thought I could! I thought I could!"; and we learned the alphabet and how to count in both languages, and on sunny days we would grab a plastic bag of leftover bread and drive over to the man-made lake at the Junkersdorfer Stadium, settle ourselves at the edge of the water, rip our stash into pieces and toss it to the skitterish little ducks and the long-necked swans floating contentedly in place.

And we sang. Teddy Ruxpin was a favorite, but this singing bear came in second to Marc's favorite song sung by Whitney Houston, "Saving All My Love for You." I'd sit on the floor in front of the stereo cabinet and start to sing with him and when he sensed that that special part was nearing, he urgently patted my shoulder, "No! No! Let me sing it, Mommy," he'd say, whereupon he'd continue singing along barely above a whisper, "I-got-to-get-ready-just-a-few-minutes-more" until he got to his favorite part and hammered home "TONIGHT is the NIGHT! I'm feelin' AWRIGHT!" with inspired by the Holy Spirit to testify about it gesticulations, and after belting out that final "youuuuuu" falsetto at the end of the song, he'd shout out "*Nochmals*, (again) Mommy!"

Occasionally, if I had a run to make and it would just be easier to leave Marc at home, Jutta, a teenager who lived a couple blocks away would come and baby-sit. But most days he and I were pretty much glued at the hip. And it was just grand.

Overhearing Marc and me converse, people I knew on the fringes of everyday life – shopkeepers and the like, would say to me, "*Frau Mayer! Sie sollten nur Deutsch mit Ihrem Kind reden.*" ("You should only speak German with your child.") "*Nein, nein,*" I always replied. *"Er wird beide Sprachen sprechen."* ("No, no. He will speak both languages.") I couldn't express myself well enough to say that it would be downright stupid to teach him my lousy German and that it only made sense to learn the international language that just happened to be my mother tongue and that he spoke German with his father and the Germans and English with me and the Americans.

And since they, who were telling me what I should do with my kid, couldn't speak English, my kid, as a matter of fact, already had one up on them. It was frustrating that subtitles of what I really wanted to say didn't ticker tape across my forehead. But in the big picture, speaking a clear concise German was the least of my concerns. As the Germans say: *Scheiß drauf'* (translation: screw it). I liked that little ditty. Filled me with poetic inspiration.

Good grief. Now it was about to be a whole new ball game. I wasn't ready for this. His first day of kindergarten was scheduled to start in a few months. There was no way I would be allowed to stay all day and keep an eye out for him and control things. Or shall we pull up that 'p' word and say, 'pack that cotton'?

Jeez...Just when everything is going okay, why does reality have to intrude?

Well, as a parent, the bottom line is that for our children, we must aspire to move heaven and earth. So my options were zero and none. The only thing to do was to pull myself together, spit in my hands, roll up my sleeves, jump over my shadow and prepare to introduce my child to himself. My shoulders sagged.

"A sucker that ain't got no heart might as well be dead." I heard Daddy say that a thousand times. It reverberated in my ears constantly as I tried to get myself together on this issue. Wondered if me having my tail between my legs here would qualify me as one of those suckers he was talking about. My brain cells were tired. I needed a break from myself.

Five and a half months until the first day of kindergarten.

Stumped.

Staggering.

Stalling.

CHAPTER TWENTY

Woo-Hoo!

Two weeks later, March 1989. Easter. Lake Maggiore shimmered, its lakeside promenade flourished with palms, bougainvillea and magnolias, a lovely area, resplendent in luxuriant subtropical flora. This lake, the second largest in Italy and the largest in southern Switzerland, extends from the Italian-speaking part of Switzerland far into the Italian regions of Piedmont and Lombardy. The fragrance of fresh seawater, perfumed florets and comfortable warmth from the afternoon sun engulfed us and wafted up the cobbled alleys of the old town and beyond to the wooded slopes wreathing around this Swiss resort.

I sat next to Helmut on a worn wooden bench at a huge lakefront piazza crammed with cafes, restaurants, tourists and play areas for kids. Marc had just given the little "motorized" cars a break and was now taking his turn on the slide. We watched him take the stairs of the ladder one at a time, and then plop down into position, cast himself forward and with a "Woo-hoo!" enjoy his reward.

"Helmut?"

"Yeah, sweetie?"

"I think we should tell Marc now."

"You think?"

"Yes, I do. I just want to tell him and be done with it. There's no point to keep putting it off. You know we agreed to tell him before kindergarten starts so now's just as good a time as any."

"I don't know . . ."

"Well, what do you mean you don't know? We can't wait until some kid gets in his face and makes a mean remark because he can't run for long or because he has to stop to catch his breath. He has to understand a little bit about what's going on inside his little body and know that he is on the same level, if not higher than the other kids dammit!" I was on the edge of the edge.

He looked away from me. His arm grew taut around my shoulder.

"*Scheiße*," ("Shit") he said.

"I know," I sighed, patting his crossed leg.

"*Ja*, okay, okay," he said.

"Marc," I called out...in a call to courage.

He looked over towards us. "*Ja*, Mama!"

"Come here a minute, sweetie."

Helmut and I scooted opposite directions on the bench so that he could slip in between us.

"We don't have to go now, do we, Mom?"

I took a deep breath; I did not plan on coming up for air.

"No sweetie, we don't. Mommy and Papa just want to have a little talk with you for a minute. Now you know how you sometimes get out of breath and have to make a pause –"

The sun bounced off the gold in his long curly mop as he nodded his head up and down.

"...well, that happens because you have this little thing with your heart, and Mommy and Papa think you're a big enough boy now to know and understand that everybody has something because none of us is perfect–"

"Umm-hmm," he said.

"–and when kindergarten starts – are you excited?"

"*Ja!*"

"Good! Now when it starts and you meet the other kids I want you to remember that there are all kinds of interesting big people as well as little people in the world and a big part of what makes us interesting is how we are all different from each other. Just like all these pretty flowers – look how many different kinds there are. Just think, if God would have only made one kind of flower in only one color – that sure would be boring, wouldn't it?

"Umm-hmm!"

"So you're gonna see some kids who wear glasses so that they can see better, maybe you'll see some kids cry because they're scared...Some are unhappy and so they are not very nice, some are not so cute, some are fat, some are short – there's all kinds and Mama and Papa don't want you to feel bad not even for a minute because you maybe don't run as fast as some of them or if you have to slow down and make a pause because that is the way you are and there is nothing wrong with that and Papa and I love you, my handsome son."

"I love you and Papa too, pretty Mama."

"*Und Marc,*" Helmut said. "*Du sollst immer zur Mama oder mir kommen und Bescheid sagen falls jemand Dir was blödes erzählt.*" ("You should always come to Mama or me and let us know if somebody says something stupid to you.")

"*Okay Papa, mache ich.*" ("I will.")

"Cause you know Mama will be up there in a minute to kick somebody's butt!"

"Okay Mama," he giggled, tossing his head back.

It was quiet on our bench for a moment or two. Marc sat on his hands, looked straight ahead at nothing particular and dangled his legs back and forth. What was he thinking? Had I said enough? Too much? What's next? What should we do now? I didn't have long to grapple with myself before he spoke.

"Mama?"

My heart was in my throat.

"Yes, my son?"

"Can I go get back on the slide now?"

"Sure," I said.

"Woo-hoo!" he shouted out.

CHAPTER TWENTY-ONE

Always

"Mama, I love him, but he's gonna kill me! "I know it! I know it! I just want you to know it and when it happens, you can say she told –"

"Tracie, honey –"

"I swear to God, I just think it's all too much for me Mama – you know? I mean this language and this country and always worrying and now kindergarten and–"

"Okay now, calm down–"

"Sometimes I just want to come home and put my feet over the heater in the kitchen and look out at the pool and the lake and –"

"Take it easy now, take it easy and tell Mommy what happened!"

"Whew...okay...okay. Well, you know kindergarten starts day after tomorrow, right?" I extended my head above the telephone to blow my nose.

"Yes, uh-huh, uh-huh, go on!"

"So I thought we'd go shopping and pick up some little packs of juices and some snacks, you know, get ready for the big day and look for some treats for a little girl whose birthday party is at three that same afternoon—"

"What little girl?"

"Her name is Jana, you didn't meet her your last visit. I can't believe that's already been three months ago. So anyway, we were at that store on the corner of the Aachener Street, you know which corner I'm talking about – a couple blocks down the street from Maytex—"

"A couple blocks down from Maytex...Now I sure know where Helmut and the store are, but I'm not sure which corner you're talking about."

"You know, Mama! At that huge intersection where the international pharmacy is on the corner. I'm talking about the grocery store on the opposite side of that street. You went there with me!"

"Oh THAT store! Um-hmm, um-hmm, okay, okay, gotcha! So what hap...Tracie, is my grandson alright?"

"So listen Ma—"

"IS MY GRANDSON ALRIGHT?"

"Yes, Mama, he's fine, he's fine."

"Are you sure?"

"Mama, I wouldn't tell you he was fine if he wasn't fine! I'm the one with the problem!"

"Okay, okay then, go on. Wait – where is he now?"

"Upstairs in his room."

"Where are you?"

"In the basement."

"Okay, go on."

"So I – we were standing in the aisle where all the candies are and I was looking for some fruit candies and Marc was looking at the new Pez candy dispensers and the *Überraschung Eier* – you know those chocolate eggs with the little toys inside he collects and so I turn to ask him if he thought the candies I had picked out were a good choice...and he was gone."

"He was what? What do you mean he was gone?! Gone where?"

"Mama, I nearly died. I flew up and down the aisles petrified, calling out for him, and he was nowhere in sight and – all I could think was Lord, please, where is my child? Where is my child! He couldn't just vanish! Nobody could have snatched him – he would have screamed out or something and so—"

Mama gasped.

"...I took off towards the sliding glass doors at the entrance that were opened, thank God, and I swear on everything holy to me it felt like my eyes had expanded to the size of saucers in my head so I could sweep the whole periphery in a shot and don't...you...know...I spotted him at first glance."

"Where was he, Tracie Lynn?"

"Mama, this kid had walked out the store to the corner, waited at the crosswalk for the green light, crossed over to the sidewalk station in the middle of the street, waited again for the signal to cross and then crossed that street over to the other sidewalk where the pharmacy is and was twirling around a street post. Singing. Head in the clouds. Just having a great time."

There was silence until Mama could catch her breath enough to inhale properly so she would have her lungs full enough to be able to split her sides laughing.

Through her tears she finally said, "What on earth would make him do that?"

"You know, Mama, I don't know HOW Marc got some crap like this in his head! I just kept my eyes on him and with the patience of Job waited on the lights and crossed over towards him. And I just kept telling myself: keep a pleasant look on your face, don't let him think you're gonna KICK HIS LITTLE BUTT WHEN YOU GET HIM IN YOUR HANDS! So when I got him into yanking-his arm-towards-me distance, I said, "Marc! Why would you leave Mommy and cross these streets by yourself? Do you know how dangerous that is?"

"And what did he say, honey?"

"I just wanted to see if I could do it, Mommy."

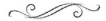

I sat sequestered in the car outside the kindergarten. Turned the ignition halfway. Radio came on. Switched it off.

"Okay, come on, now, get a grip, girlfriend," I said to myself. "Marc is safe. He is sound." The metal gates encircling the container-like building appeared to stand several head and shoulders above its flat roof.

"Yeah and he didn't hesitate the slightest when he said *"Tschüss* ("see you later") Mommy!" and turned and delightedly sashayed off into a room splashed with color and cutouts, miniature tables and chairs...damn it."

I had previously discussed his medical situation with his two teachers, Betty and Sabine. "Don't worry," they assured me. "We'll keep an eye out for him, he'll be fine." A pat on the arm and the reiterated assurance again today. I felt so proud, so accomplished, so damn miserable.

"How could Mama and Daddy let me leave and go to Europe?! If Marc ever pulls a stunt on me like that I'll wring his neck."

Well, I could either remain parked here stewing behind the steering wheel and take the risk that someone would peek out from behind a young master's painted, scissored and posted window vignette and catch me sniveling or I could speed home and sit by the telephone. It would only take me five minutes to get back here.

"I feel so secure when we're together. How on this sweet earth am I going to cut the umbilical cord?"

"By the looks of things, you may have to probably reinvent yourself, ol' gal."

"Yeah, okay fine and dandy! Into what?"

"I don't know what you want to call it – but today you've taken the first step. A major step. How do they say it? Loving is letting go and encouraging wings to..."

"You can just shut that bullshit right up because I know just as good as I'm sitting here I am going to without exception invoke all my rights as his mother to whoop and wail, shout and scream, and howl and yowl with full lungs to the world until I forfeit the right which will never happen –"

"How do you know you won't forfeit the right by going on the poor kid's nerves?"

"I'll tell you why, because neither one of us can make a U-turn on our contract – that's why. And if it seems that I'm all agog, well that's probably because I am and I defy anybody to get in my way, and you know what –?"

"Inner being to woman behind the steering wheel...Am I detecting a slight slipping of our sanity?"

"MAYBE! But no matter! Let me break this down for you so you will have no "uh-ruhs" as daddy used to say when the dummies didn't 'get it'. I am basically just a straight-ahead decent kind o' girl and I am not too damn demented to know that I'm not offering Marc Utopia – not even by a long shot – but this is me and that's just the cross he will have to bear 'cause I'm always gonna be his Mama. Neurotic or not. And that's just the way it is, and the way it will be."

Always.

Always.

Always.

I turned the key and started the ignition.

"Marc came at four years old into the kindergarten. He was in the 'Schweinchengruppe' ('Little Piglet Group'). Despite his heart illness he was a bright, happy and self-confident child. After we explained to the children about Marc's illness,

they and the other teachers dealt with it simply as a matter of course. Despite his physical weakness, he showed strength and courage toward his environment. For example, he would raise a flexed arm and say, 'I'm the strongest!' Like every other child he was liked and accepted. His illness was not a disadvantage in kindergarten."

~Betty and Sabine, Kindergarten teachers

CHAPTER TWENTY-TWO

Trusting the Body

You are not prepared for the bells that jingle jangle as if through a megaphone when you push open the front door, nor the infectious kinetic energy that bowls you over precisely the moment you step inside. Your eyes widen in wonder and anticipation.

Sensual reggae rhythms pulsate from somewhere at the top of the staircase – instantly knocking that uptight 'I've never been here before' edge off – and you soon realize that the soulful syncopation furnishes the backdrop for a steady stream of fusing voices. Invigorated and inviting. Laughing. High-fiving. Distinguished accents from the Islands, Americas, Africa, and Europe. An acoustical panorama of the world. You get a hunch that you won't be the only one trying to suppress the impulse to nod on the downbeat and when snapping your fingers, and when unabashed sporadic vocal accompaniments chime in within earshot – you feel like...like you've finally broken through the constrictions and the gates have been thrown open for you to make a communal connection!

Say Zeebra Tropicana and you say open sesame.

Rooted in the hub of the city of Cologne, this hair salon offers umpteen hair-styling products and everything from facial hair remover to Ghanaian plantains. It seems to be an event unto itself, reflected in its patronage which ranges from the *hoi polloi* to the hoity-toity. The place is bursting at the seams with people – sometimes all day long. For me, it was love at first sight and where I had the good fortune of meeting Rupert Shonaike, master in Chinese self-defense, calisthenics and Course Leader of the Tai Chi Studio of Cologne.

He had been standing near the front desk and had a bird's-eye view of Marc and me holding hands, making our slow ascent of the ten stairs from the entrance door. Once we reached the top landing, his gaze zeroed in on Marc.

When she isn't styling hair, Baaba, the proprietress of the salon, weaves about, stringing people together, engaging this one and that in conversation. She'll try to find a lid for every pot; because this proud Ghanaian Christian woman, who quickly became my dear friend, firmly believes that by helping each other we ultimately help ourselves. And she sets forth about this as if on a mission.

She introduced Rupert to Marc and me.

During the course of our conversation, this gentle man explained to me that the practice of Tai Chi Chuan, the ancient Chinese system of exercise, has both self-defense and meditative connotations in that it increases blood circulation, strengthens muscles, eases tension and calms the heart. He didn't have to say another word, but he went on.

"It would help Marc to find a good way of breathing and balancing himself," he said. "Breathing quietly would help him to learn to trust his body, you see, because he'd have more physical confidence, coordination and control."

Confidence, coordination and control. As essential for my son as reading, writing and 'rithmatic.

He had me hanging on every word when he at last explained that the movements are gentle, done in an even slow tempo and synchronized with one's own breathing.

Marc had his first one-hour lesson the following week. Needless to say I was smiling from ear to ear not only because of the very real health benefits, but also because after banging my head around trying to come up with something as an alternative to standard sports and continually coming up empty-handed, I'd finally hit the jackpot. Marc looked forward to his twice weekly one-on-one session and with first grade on the horizon, I had one less major concern because now he too would be able to pipe in with his classmates when they boasted about after-school activities. Tai Chi! As 'for boys!' and as exotic sounding as Karate! Or Judo! He had just started piano lessons, so everything was falling into place.

It was all good. It was all good.

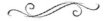

The issue just popped up. Evidently, both Helmut and I had been thinking about it because one day it just casually fell on the table. Strangely enough, neither of us had to convince the other. We could do it. And more than that, we wanted to do it. We were unconquerable – after all, during the six years we'd been married, we'd actually built a picket fence on stable grounds – grounds that paved over the obstacle courses that encircled our little family. So why not?

There was a snag.

Firmly rooted in my brain, agitating the chemicals therein, it ran the length of my body, transmitting disruptive signals, but because month after month I had my menstrual cycle, I was unaware that I'd been thrown off balance, left without issue...fallow. I had a total aversion to the uninvited guest that antagonized me. But we had grown accustomed to each other for so long that one couldn't avoid the other and eventually, my co-tenant got comfortable to the point of just outright taking over my body and turning it against itself. The ultimate double cross to any woman with my intentions.

But aside from this factor of chronic stress, another element had infested my brain, and settled itself like the plague, deeper than bone in my body. It was the undercurrent compelling my contentment to remain at low ebb.

I needed an answer, expert confirmation...one way or the other.

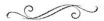

Dear Colleague Tinschman,

Mr. And Mrs. Mayer would like to have a child. Due to the complex heart defect of their only child thus far, they are now inquiring about the risk of a repetition...

...this syndrome in the vast majority of cases occurs sporadically...however, there are several families described in which siblings had the disease...

The patient would in case of the birth of another child be at least thirty-four years old, if not thirty-five. At thirty-four she has a risk of 0.4% for a chromosomally diseased child, at thirty-five that risk would increase to about 1%. With the aid of an amniotic fluid puncture one can admittedly not diagnose a heart defect...

Should another pregnancy occur, which I can only recommend, I would be very grateful for the notification of the infant's data.

Pediatrician, Medicinal Geneticist, Cologne, February, 1990

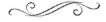

...Well, I guess I really didn't want any more babies, after all. Actually that's a lie. But after my visit with the geneticist, I would have to admit that in a sense, I was relieved. Even though we were encouraged to extend our family from well-wishers, family and medical professionals alike, the truth is – and I'm no longer ashamed to admit it – I couldn't conquer my own fear. Point blank. Shoot me dead. Couldn't do it. Even when I thought I was calm, panic would slurp up my inner senses and spit them far out into a gulf beset with peril.

And it goes without saying that if some kind of divine inspiration couldn't help me, Helmut didn't have a chance. Assistance from anyone would have not only been futile, but intrusive, because, though I was confounded by many things, of one thing I was certain. This truth resonated within the chamber of my very soul: The manuscript of our lives is not signed with our own individual signature. What is it they say about telling God your plans? I didn't believe in crystal gazing and knew I wouldn't have the stamina to stroke a rabbit's foot for nine months and would have undoubtedly driven Helmut out of his mind with my jitters.

This malady, though sporadic, could happen again. There was no guarantee that I would have a baby born free of disease. This was just the little bundle of informatics I needed. It of course rode along well with the perfect excuse to cover up or excuse my angst to myself: "It's not me incompetent and unproductive crying quits – it's them! Those sluggish-ass ovaries! It's their fault I can't have another baby!" Shifting the blame served only to reinforce the twisted alignment of my brain with my body for it didn't take a halo of illumination to realize that no matter where I tossed the ball, it was still in my court. Helmut, forever the optimist, had no reservations, or if he did, he never let on. I don't think he could have realized or understood the depths of my fear and I didn't want him to – I mean, what's with all the phobia? I'm made of sterner stuff than that!

So my psychopathic mental self-slaughter remained a private matter. I was fed up with myself and filled with contempt that I was so damn sniveling and pathetic that I just couldn't pull myself together. I was sure of something else which was that I alone could heal myself and only through thought. I often recalled the times, perplexed about one thing or another, I would seek Daddy's advice and he would proclaim, "You got to get your mind right!" Well, I was nowhere near there yet, and as far as this issue was concerned, I probably never would be – there. Kind of like once bitten, twice shy. And good, bad or ugly, that's just the way it was.

It took some serious soul-searching, but I eventually justified my inability to conceive by telling myself that sometimes one must leave well enough alone. What may seem puzzling does indeed have intended design. What else was there?

Helmut and I didn't share our disappointment with anyone other than ourselves, but there was no perpetual blurring of the eyes or overwhelming sense of loss for that second crop that lay somewhere over the hills far away from us. No, no. We had too much to be thankful for in our particular little cul-de-sac; we three still had each other and that was our four corners of the world.

CHAPTER TWENTY-THREE

Is it Them or Me?

Three weeks before the first day of Marc's entering first grade, he and I were hospitalized for three days at the Cologne University Clinic. We had a room to ourselves, Marc now had a full-sized bed, and I slept next to it on a cot on the floor. Compared to previous visits, this wasn't nearly as bad. Though the room was bare of any amenities and the toilet and washing facilities were down the hall, we at least had our privacy.

The cardiac catheterization took place because of a rise in the hemoglobin level to over 18%, the question being whether and if so, what kind of operative measures would be possible...to improve pulmonary perfusion.

...in consultation with our cardiac surgeon: because of the high pressure values on the right side of the lung, it would be out of the question to conduct a Fontan or Glenn operation...

If further palliative measures are possible...then the result of the cardiac catheterization check forbids a so-called "functional" correction of the cardiac defect according to the Fontan method.

The Professor, 13 August, 1991

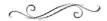

Upon our discharge, the Professor instructed me to get Marc's blood count every three to six months and to keep him abreast of how things were going. Furthermore, he indicated that Marc could be excused from school sports as he wished; he indeed knew his limits and would participate accordingly. As far as the necessity of another operation, arrangements should be made for Helmut and me to confer with the hospital's recently appointed director of heart surgery.

I had a lot to think about before the first day of school.

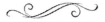

Two weeks after school started, we sat down with the surgeon.

Dear Professor,

Marc Mayer's parents requested an interview and I would like to report to you about the course of the conversation...

At the most recent examination in our joint conference...We were in total agreement that a corrective operation was out of the question and even a definitive palliation after modification of the Fontan procedure could not be considered...

I proposed as the next step to emplace a Glenn anastomosis...currently a surgical procedure is not necessary...possibly within the next six months.

The child is in your care, the parents will get back to you.

Director and University Professor of Heart Surgery, Clinic of Cologne, September 25, 1991

Helmut and I were absolutely not in agreement, nothing could have been further from the truth – however the surgeon had done his best to convince us that we had no other options.

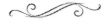

Sometime during the first weeks of school on a glorious autumn day, the first graders and the mothers who could attend set out on the first class field trip. The meeting point was a woodsy area not too far from the school.

We started our journey at a comfortable pace on a lonely path that sloped and dipped and seemed to stretch on forever. Gradually the momentum picked up and the kids, one after the other, then the moms were galloping behind the teacher toward wherever we were headed, so I swooped Marc up in my arms, settled him on my hip and hippity-hopped along. We reached our destination with a few couldn't waiters pulling up before us and others bringing up the rear.

A huge field unfolded before us, golden in the daylight, at its center could've been a monstrous stack of hay or a mountain of beetroots, I don't remember. Marc sprang from my arms and joined his classmates in idle play. I watched him, and trailed not too far behind. My stance didn't reveal the fact that no! things were not just fine and that while earnestly observing the setting, my thoughts were snarled up with questions like: How well would my son be able to keep up with and fit in with these zippity-zing kids? Are they a decent bunch? Who here would prove to be the class bully?

Jesus, the stairs.

How will Marc master going up and down forty-odd stairs several times a day, particularly when the first and the last bells of the day ring out and he's got to bear the weight of his Scout book bag on his back? Why couldn't the school just have regular desks with writing tables that lift up and reveal storage space for the books and papers and crayons and ink and all the crap these first graders didn't need to carry home to study with every night? Is he really going to have to have another operation? Is all this school stuff going to exacerbate that necessity?

Did I remember to let the office secretary know to inform the school principal about Marc? I'm sure I did...didn't I? Think hard...what was it she said? Did I write down the telephone number where Helmut could be reached during the day? What about Dr. Tinschman's...and Mama's – in case I get hit by a car while running an errand and Helmut passes out under the weight of a carpet roll?

Over time, living tense and on guard, had rendered me quick on my feet, so you can imagine how I felt when his teacher quietly eased up, positioned herself within close range and knocked me out with a left hook.

"*Es ist ein wunderschönen Tag Heute,*" she said.

"Yes, it is a very nice day," I replied in German, smiling, grateful she had inadvertently given me the opportunity to seize the moment to remind her to keep an extra eye out for my son. Marc would be attending this *Grundschule* (elementary school) for four years primarily under her tutelage, which meant his morning to midday custodial care would be in her hands, so needless to say I would be eternally grateful to know that she would maintain a protective lookout for my son.

"It must be very difficult for you to see the other children running while your child can't," she said.

"Huh?" I thought and did a double take. No doubt I looked like I'd swallowed another one of those stupid pills.

I knew that she herself had children and at that very moment, I asked myself, if one of them had been born blind, how she would feel if someone had said, "It must be difficult to watch the other children creating beautiful crafts while your child gropes about in the darkness." I nodded and sort of smiled, though I didn't feel smiley, and continued to follow the silver haired schoolmarm who was again skipping and singing through a field in the middle of nowhere. As I looked at her, I couldn't help but to wonder, what, just what on this sweet earth did she expect me to say?

It was moments like this when I wondered: Is it them...or me?

Things have a way of working themselves out.

In the mornings, after seeing Marc inside the enclosed gates of the school grounds, I discreetly, (tried to be anyway), carried his school bag up the stairs and left it sitting outside the classroom door and scurried back to my car. After school, sometimes, one of his classmates would carry the bag back down. This relieved me greatly. I couldn't be the only mom hovering outside the classroom door at the close of every school day. It was reassuring to see that Marc was capable of handling his situation and not afraid to accept help.

Marc told me many years later, that he did get harassed and teased from some of his classmates, both because of the color of his skin and his heart ailment. I wish he had told me. At the time, he only mentioned one class bully who was particularly troubling to him. This boy was almost two years older than the others in the class and who, probably because of his own insecurities, made fun of everyone, so his remarks about Marc's health and skin color are unmemorable. Upon speaking with his mother, one could only consider the bottom of the barrel source. Let it suffice to say that after our confrontation, there were no more slides directed at my son from hers.

On more than one occasion after school started, I would sit down with Marc and explain to him that "It's more important what you have up here," pointing at my temple, "than what you have here," pointing at my flexed bicep. Helmut always reinforced this. At this rough and tumble time of his young life, I thought it critical to develop and maintain a clear distinction between the brains and brawn thing, to let him know he didn't have to fight with his fists, that real strength lay in his ability to think and in his character. Especially in light of the fact that I thought he was starting to breathe heavier.

CHAPTER TWENTY-FOUR

Here We Go Again

By February of 1992, I was sure of it. The previous December, lukewarm baths and thoughts of Santa coming to town helped him get through an attack of the chicken pox. On January 9, 1992 he came down with a fever, but strangely enough, had no telltale signs of any illness. Four days later he had a crowding tooth extracted and took antibiotics a few days as a hedge against infection, which lent me a bit of relief, certain as I was that this buffer would serve equally well as a bane to whatever was giving rise to his elevated temperature.

Six days later his temperature rose again and Dr. Tinschman prescribed another antibiotic. This prescription ran its course by the end of January. Sometime during the first week in February, we were issued another antibiotic and after several days of waiting it out, Marc and I were again in Dr. Tinschman's office.

"I'm not leaving here until you figure out why this fever won't break," I said.

"*Ich verstehe das nicht,*" he said, frowning, propping Marc up on the examination table.

"I don't understand it either!" I said, my fingers frantically pulling Marc's sweater over his head and nearly ripping away the buttons on his shirt to get at his undershirt so the stethoscope could be pressed against his chest.

"I've given him his medicines just like I was supposed to and his temperature gets a little lower, but before long, it starts—"

The stethoscope moved from here to there. I shut my mouth so Dr. Tinschman wouldn't miss anything.

After a few moments, he removed the apparatus from his ears, draped it around his neck, turned and moved towards his desk a few feet away from the examination bed. I knew he was headed for the telephone. A fifty-fifty sense of exhilaration and apprehension rapidly spiraled from my feet up my body, instantly swelling in my head: finally we were going to get to the bottom of this – but what would it entail?

"I'm going to make arrangements for you to take him to the University Clinic now," he said, picking up the telephone receiver and dialing the number. "I don't know what he has, but he must go into the hospital and be intensively checked. Immediately."

And so it was. An hour and a half later, Marc and I checked back into 'our' room. And there we stayed from February 12 until March 22.

During the first two days, at varying intervals, four blood cultures were made. Before the results of the first cultures came in, Marc was set up on an intravenous antibiotic therapy. A few days passed. A conversation with the Hygiene Institute confirmed that the cultures revealed a bacterial infection, but no one could pinpoint just what it was. Though he continued the original intravenous therapy thereafter in conjunction with a second antibiotic, Marc remained feverish, the doctors stumped and Helmut and me doing our best to hold on in the maelstrom.

Several more days passed and finally, the Institute confirmed the cause of Marc's malaise: endocarditis; an infection of the heart's inner lining caused by bacteria. I wondered if the chicken pox had anything to do with this. Though the varicella virus is a common infection in children, complications can and do occur, the most prominent being a bacterial infection of the sore itself, particularly if scratched. I really didn't know what introduced this particular pathogen into Marc's bloodstream, but if it wasn't immediately eliminated, it could kill him.

After that last conversation with the Hygiene Institute, the medication he was initially given was switched over to an intravenous penicillin, which he took together with that same second antibiotic for another two weeks. Aside from these megadosages of chemical substances, he swallowed a cough medicine and inhaled saltwater three and four times a day respectively.

I kept steadfast notes of his temperature, the medicines, the amounts and the times when he took them. I never gave any thought to what I was doing; it was just my way of staying on top of the situation as I'd always done. It was my security blanket as well as a form of control – I didn't have to ask someone what was what when. One might think that my notes (though no one ever knew exactly what it was I wrote down) and uninterrupted observations of Marc and remarks or questions would be considered a help to the staff – certainly not a hindrance.

Not that it matters; hindsight is irrelevant to the moment as it happens anyway. The bottom line was to see to it that my child was healed. Each passing minute this thing was not arrested, Marc's life fell deeper in jeopardy. So if my behavior kept them at the apex of their job performance, then so be it. So be it very well. I soon came to realize that my being in the thick of things, more than likely, contributed to the doctors on duty being more formal with me than pleasant. There's contortion for you: They had the nerve to give me wary looks when they were the ones reading my son's chart and scratching their heads.

And then one day, they learned the extent of my watch and ward. One of the head doctors in particular. The Professor was making his late afternoon rounds and, as he did a couple of times a day, checked in on Marc. He and three or four doctors stood clustered near the foot of Marc's bed, conferring with one another. I rose up from my chair next to Marc, and with opened notebook and pen in hand, joined them.

"So he does appear to be improving."

"Yes, Professor, his temperature has not broken, but it is steadily falling," the head doctor, said.

The Professor looked over the chart. "So when was the last time you gave him the Mucolyse?"

My eyes darted to my notes. The *Oberärztin* (head doctor) tossed her hair over her shoulder and from her incredible memory started rattling off her account of things.

I looked at her sharply, frowned and shook my head.

"Frau Mayer, is something incorrect?" the Professor asked. I was unaware that he'd been observing me.

"That's not right what she said," I said, as I scanned the day's entries in my little notebook. "At 11:30 he was given 30 milliliters of the Mucolyse and then he did the inhalation." I stepped closer towards the Professor, held the notebook open under his nose before he even had a chance to mutter, "That is not necessary," and indexed with my finger along the page what time what took place. I could feel his eyes following my finger as I went along. "At 12:15 his temperature was still 38.5," I said looking up at him to make sure he was with me. "At one o'clock he was given the Penicillin with the Refobacin. That was over two hours ago.

"You can read it yourself," I said, thrusting my little book of notes and charts into his hands.

His eyebrows converged and stayed that way as he slowly turned the pages. If Mama had been in the room there with us, she'd have leaned towards me and mouthed, "It's so quiet you can hear a mouse piss on cotton." Suddenly, for some inexplicable reason I began to feel self-conscious. My gaze fell to the floor. Maybe I'd spot that mouse. Though no more than a couple minutes at most, it seemed an eternity for the Professor to finish reading my notes. My focal point drifted to Marc. He was staring at me. I winked. He winked back. The quiet continued to simmer.

My gaze shifted over to the solitary window. It's thick multi-paned glass divided the dull gray daylight passing into the room. This was the kind of dreary day that normally would render the townspeople poker-faced with suitably associated dispositions, but outside at this very minute, the folks of this city were shedding their buttoned-up, zipped-up state of control to the bareness of complete and utter self-abandonment as one of the wildest carnival experiences to be had in Europe was riotously getting into full swing.

It all officially begins on the 11th day of the 11th month at 11 minutes past the 11th hour smack dab in the center of the *Altermarkt* (Old Market), a square located in the middle of the historical old city. The balloons and the streamers go up at about the same time the Christmas trees come down, but watch out! Today is *Weiberfastnacht!* (Women's Carnival), the day that sets off a week of outrageous festivities with impromptu street parties and people in every kind of costume imaginable – the more colorful and crazy the better – and the old and the young, friends and strangers alike will greet one another with *Prosit* (toasts) to their beloved city with shouts of *Kölle Alaaf!* (Cologne above all!) and businesses will close early and it won't be long before the Brauhäuser and pubs will be filled to overflowing with glitzy tipsy patrons locking arms and *schaukeln* (swaying) from side to side, singing the carnival songs and there will be endless balls and beer and kisses and on Rose Monday the granddaddy of all the city's parades will see well over a million people in the streets and then finally by Ash Wednesday, the restaurants will be packed with pooped partiers back in their everyday garb eating fish and lamenting that on *"Asche Mittwoch ist alles vorbei."* (Ash Wednesday it's all over)

And we three would be sitting at our regular table in our favorite restaurant just around the corner from our house and in between bites of trout, we'd laugh at what the natives had worn and what they daringly hadn't worn and I just know that Marc would've wanted to be a Ninja Turtle this year. Last year, he donned the cape and mask of the friendly crusader Batman and the year before that he was a pirate...and the year he was Charlie Chaplin, he looked so doggone adorable. He was all but swallowed up in a pair of fossilized trousers Helmut dug out from the back of his closet and—"

"Frau Mayer," the Professor said holding my notebook out towards me. His voice didn't reach my ears.

"Frau Mayer," he said, this time a bit louder.

"Oh! Yes!" I said snapping back to the matter at hand. *"Verzeihung,"* ("Pardon me") I said, taking my book from him.

"Danke," he said to me. "Thank you. Everything's clear."

He looked at his head doctor. He didn't yell. He didn't show his fury if indeed he was infuriated. His voice sounded, in fact, like it was held in a tight grasp.

"You would serve yourself better to go celebrate carnival and leave Frau Mayer here to do your work."

And with that he turned, opened the door and walked out of the room.

CHAPTER TWENTY-FIVE

Little Hans

You know, my take on things wasn't complicated: As long as Marc had to stay in the hospital, I intended to give him as much of a sense of normalcy as possible, which meant continuing on with his twice-weekly piano lessons and being tutored so that he wouldn't fall behind in his schoolwork. Easy. Nothing difficult about it. Though he was hooked up to an intravenous tube, he was capable of stimulating his mind with more than just his Gameboy. I couldn't allow that "I'm sick, I can't work, woe is so pity me" attitude to slip up on either one of us.

Helmut brought a keyboard to the room and some of Marc's music books so he could practice. His music teacher was an angel. Normally I drove Marc to her studio but to accommodate our circumstances, she made arrangements to come to the hospital and give him his lessons.

I wasn't so lucky with the hospital tutor whose approach to instructing Marc absolutely interfered with my theory of the universe. Just to show you how small the world is, I eventually found out that she actually lived down the block from us. If I'd known that it was her living room window painted over with the bug-eyed face of a woman with long nervous blond hair smiling down onto a street sign that pointed towards the *Friedhof* (cemetery), and if I'd known that it was her car painted purple with odd-sized yellow stars jumping all over it beforehand, I'd have saved myself a shouting match.

The first day she came in she seemed to be pleasant enough.

"*Guten Tag*," she said after knocking and peeping around the door. Marc, fully dressed and sitting on his bed, and I had been expecting her.

"Hello," I said standing up and heading towards her.

"I am Tracie Mayer and this is my son, Marc."

"Good day," she said again. "I am Frau Lorbach, the private teacher," she said, accepting my extended hand.

She flashed a big wide-gapped tooth smile towards Marc, now standing beside his bed, then walked over towards him and shook his free hand.

"So, you're Marc," she said taking a seat on the side of the bed.

Well, this is working out just fine, I remember thinking. She seems friendly enough and working here at the hospital as tutor primarily to young children, she'll no doubt know exactly what to instruct Marc in and how to go about it. I breathed a sigh of relief.

I picked up and carried my chair over to the opposite side of the room and settled down with page sixty-four of the novel I'd been reading. The private teacher and student got warmed up with a little chit-chat, then finally started to get down to the meat of the matter. Frau Lorbach pulled a large-print picture book out of her bag and started reading, inviting Marc to participate by looking at the pictures, responding (I guess) to the intonations in her voice and answering her questions.

"So now, why do you suppose the little boy didn't want to cross the street?" This little exchange went on for twenty minutes. Then she slid the book back into her bag and slipped her jacket back on. She'd return day after tomorrow, she said.

I looked up from page sixty-four. "What? That's all?" I said.

"Frau Mayer, we don't want to overwork the children. Like I said, I'll be back day after tomorrow." She spoke to me as if I were a young pup, contented with a little pat on the head.

Maybe she knew something I didn't so I left it at that. We'd see what would happen day after tomorrow. Lunch was more than a good hour away, and Marc had already practiced his keyboard. I looked at him. He eyed me with the look of a chess player a move away from checkmate. Puckered lips could not repress thoughts of 'what a joke!' causing the corners of his mouth to turn up.

He shrugged his shoulders and said "Well, Mama," and in the same breath began to whistle a little jive and bobbed his curly little head to its rhythm, while proceeding to carefully maneuver the intravenous tube around himself as he crawled up and plopped down on his bed, crossed his legs beneath him, swooped his Gameboy out from underneath his pillow, and then, giggly all the way down to his fingertips, settled back into his down filled cushion. He and Super Mario would face off against the elements until lunchtime.

I walked over and picked up my chair. I couldn't suppress my own smile. "You know what I used to tell your granddaddy, Marc?" I said as I set my seat back in place and sat down next to him. His eyes remained riveted on his game as he said, "What Mama?"

"You can't bullshit a bullshitter and that goes for you too!"

He guffawed and said, "Mama, you are so funny!"

Two days later, the same thing happened. I couldn't believe she was getting paid for this. After thirty minutes she gathered up her things and gaily told Marc, "See you day after tomorrow!" Marc said, "*Tschüss!*" ("Bye-bye!") and exchanged glances with me. I didn't have to open my mouth for him to comprehend that he'd better stop looking at me like this whole thing was just a laugh a minute.

This clearly wasn't working for me. I accompanied her to the door. Once outside in the hallway I expressed my concern. Maybe my approach was wrong – but I really had neither the time nor patience to pussyfoot around. Experience had shown me that when confronted with a problem, tackle it and get it out of the way, so that the center of intellect is not punch drunk when the time comes – and believe me, it will come – to focus on the next irritation.

"Frau Lorbach, is this all you plan to do with Marc, just read to him, because if so, you don't need to trouble yourself. I can do that myself," I said.

"Frau Mayer, as I told you, we don't want to overwork the children."

"Overwork him? Wait a minute! What's he doing? You're not teaching him anything! The whole point of your being here is to work with him, teach him what he'd be learning if he were in school right now – you know, like Math and German and how to write and whatever else it is kids in the first grade in the German public school system learn. I don't want him to fall behind the class. I thought you would give him some homework, something constructive to do that he would have to give you to be corrected –"

"Frau Mayer! The child is ill! You cannot –"

"Frau...Frau..." Her name had escaped me. "First of all, please do not tell me what I can and cannot do with my child. I know him. I know his strengths and his weaknesses and yes! he does have an infection and yes! he is being strongly medicated and yes! he is getting better and yes! I am doing all I can to make him have a sense of a normal day cooped up here in this hospital!

And if he's fit enough to practice his piano every day and get Super Mario from the lowest to the highest level, then he's surely fit enough to get something constructive in his head and asking him why little Hans didn't want to cross the street is not gonna get it!"

At this point she started walking hastily away from me, but I just figured she was in a hurry, so I sped up and walked right along beside her down the corridor.

"You don't understand – the child is sick!" she said.

"I KNOW that! So what should I do? Say "Oh, you poor child, you are so sick?" Because if that's what you think then think again because I will not do that! It doesn't even come into consideration. I have to make this child see that he is getting better every day – and he is! He's got to get it in his head that this is just a temporary little setback – that it could happen to anybody and things are not all that bad and just to prove it to himself he needs to practice his music every day and he needs to do some schoolwork every day with the expectation that quite soon he will be back home and things will be fine again.

"But I need your help. I am Marc's mother, his friend, his playmate and I teach him what I can – but I cannot do it all! And I shouldn't have to – you are supposed to be the teacher here, and I expect you to present him with a planned course of study of the appropriate subject matter. Is that so difficult to understand?"

A nurse scuttled past us into the open door of the nurses' station. "Look," I said. "It's just like when the nurse comes to take his temperature, I expect her to bring a thermometer – not a buttered *Brötchen*. I don't want to insult you but this is really not complicated! And we certainly don't have to argue about it!" I slowed to a standstill as she continued down the hallway. "Frau Mayer," she said over her shoulder, "I think the best is for me to speak with the Professor. I'm sure—"

"You're sure what? You think the Professor can straighten me out here?" She rounded the bend of the hallway, heading for the stairs and briskly clicked the heels of her ankle boots down onto the landing.

"After I talk to him about this you may have to get some other books to put in your bag there!" I yelled down over the stair railing.

"You know what, Frau Mayer?" she called out, "I won't be back!"

"Hey! You know what else, Frau...Private teacher? Fine! The few minutes that you're here are just a waste of time anyway!" I said.

If it looks like a duck and acts like a duck, it probably is a duck, but there ain't no givin' up and no givin' out.

I made a call to the school. Luckily, Marc's teacher knew of a young man studying to become an elementary school teacher and who would be happy to tutor Marc and earn some extra money. I had him bring the books that the class was using at the time so Marc felt a part of the group even though he wasn't physically there. And by the time he did go back to class, those feelings of being left out and having fallen behind were not an issue. This no doubt did wonders for his self-esteem. I mean, the problem was not that daunting.

Funny how when things work out, we never take the time to stop and consider that they work out...

And so, life went on. On clear nights I'd always make the same wish upon the brightest star.

We traveled by plane, (Marc never experienced any difficulty with the three or four hour flights), by car and by rail in Europe. The basics of Marc's medical reports were translated into English, Spanish and French. These documents – all of them – were without exception tucked away inside the family pharmacy bag, which except for when I was sleeping, was always hanging from my shoulder during our holidays.

Marc carried on with school, Tai Chi and his music lessons. Sometime in his third school year, his classmates started swimming lessons once a week. I enrolled Marc and myself in a parent-child evening swim course for physically challenged children. After a few visits, Marc decided he didn't need the extra classes. Unbelievably, he took to the water like a fish and earned his swimming certificate right alongside the rest of his classmates.

Still, I often longed for breezy thoughts.

Not a single day went by that I didn't worry.

CHAPTER TWENTY-SIX

Nirvana

I kicked the covers away the morning of January 5, 1994 in a state of premonition panic. The moment I'd been dreading was now at hand. Marc had grown progressively weaker over the last months, more short of breath. The Professor would be waiting for us at eleven o'clock. He would confirm my worst fears. I just knew it. Didn't matter that my soul screamed itself scarlet, there was nothing I could do but stand up to reality and face it.

The checkup completed, Marc was popping his head back into his undershirt. The Professor and I sat at opposite sides of the examination table.

"So have there been any particular observations lately?" the Professor said.

"Well, you know, I think that his breathing is getting heavier and that he looks bluer underneath his eyes and on his fingertips," I said. "And he makes longer pauses when walking. He also told me that he got dizzy for a moment or two a couple times at school. He's never said that before."

"Um-hmm." He paused, and then sighed. "Well, his oxygen levels today are between 77 and 81 percent," he said, leafing through a stack of papers from Marc's file. "His shunts sound good, but his hemoglobin values do appear to be steadily rising. I don't think we have to do anything right now, but the time is coming when we will have to decide..."

"Well, what means right now? How much time do we have?"

"That I can't say," he said. "It could be soon, very soon, or it could be a month or two or maybe six months from now. It's hard to say, but I think that we must be prepared."

"Well, what kind of operation will the surgeon want to do?" I said.

He looked at me, and then his gaze dropped to the table. He looked over at Marc now busily buttoning his shirt. "I don't know. We won't know until we open him up."

That was the wrong answer. It went way, way beyond the pale of my understanding.

He continued talking, but he might as well have spoken to the four walls for I had once again left the room. My mind had a tendency to do that when certain utterances stung my senses. I remember thinking: If this man thinks even for a nanosecond that I'm letting somebody cut open my child based upon a procedure called Let's Wait and See Until He's Lying There with His Chest Cavity Carved Open and Leaking, he must be out of his last mind. If he wants a guinea pig he'd better go get a damn hamster.

Maybe I said something. Maybe I didn't.

The floor was hard as granite beneath my feet. I don't remember saying good-bye. But I know I didn't vacillate as I gripped Marc's hand as we left the building.

A couple days later, Helmut drove to the city of Hanover for the international carpet fair. He would be there for two days. During that time I had an appointment with my gynecologist for my half yearly pap smear, for Kasimir our Yorkshire Terrier to go to the vet to get his teeth cleaned and for Marc to get his DPT shot and then attend Lydia's birthday party. That still left me too much time to crawl up inside myself and implode. I told Helmut I'd go to the store in between all my running around and keep an eye out on things.

I took a seat that Wednesday afternoon several feet away from the front desk. Close enough to hear what was going on, yet far enough away not to be disturbed. I pulled an issue of Good Housekeeping magazine from my purse. Mama had read this magazine for years and I picked up her habit. I bought this issue at the train station, the only place I knew at the time that sold an array of American magazines. Flipping through the pages, I came upon an insert, a booklet actually, and got a jolt. The title said "The 400 BEST DOCTORS IN AMERICA". I quickly turned the pages to Cardiac Surgery. Underneath the headline it stated: "These specialists operate on the heart and its blood vessels; some also operate on the lungs and other organs of the chest."

I decided to write to two of these surgeons: Dr. Aldo Castañeda, because it said in brackets after his name and Children's Hospital, Boston, Massachusetts: congenital problems, 90% of patients are children. And the other doctor was Dr. Albert Starr, of St. Vincent's Hospital, in Portland, Oregon. I chose him because Oregon neighbors my home state. In the event he could help us, my family members would be nearby.

Dear Dr. –

My name is Tracie Frank Mayer. I am an American living in Cologne, West Germany. I have read in an American magazine that you have been named as one of the outstanding heart surgeons in America. I have therefore, forwarded my son's medical reports to you in the hopes that you can, if you will, with this limited information, give me your opinion.

At this time, Marc is nine years old. As you can see in the medical reports, he has had two palliative surgeries. With his hemoglobin values rising the past years (now between 18 and 19.8) and his oxygen saturation values between 77 and 81, the doctors here in Cologne believe the time is again approaching for us to once again prepare for surgery.

With this limited information here, Dr. – is it possible that you could suggest a particular operative procedure that would be beneficial to my son?

I am sincerely grateful for your time and attention, and a healthy happy new year from my family to yours,
    Tracie, January 14, 1994

Along with this letter I sent copies of the cardiology report from Professor Bourgeois, the December 5, 1985 report from the surgeon who performed Marc's second operation and the May 8, 1987 report from the Professor at the Cologne Clinic. I had absolutely nothing and yet somehow everything to lose. So, now all I could do was wait and see. And pray. Because you never know...

January 20, 1994, I received a letter. It read in part:

...Potentially he (Marc) is a candidate for what we call a Fontan reconstruction in which the arterial shunts are closed and the circulation to the lung is via a direct caval pulmonary connection...

I would suggest that you have a recent echocardiogram done and the report sent to me. Following that I will be in touch with you about whether a Fontan reconstruction is possible.
    Sincerely yours,
    Albert Starr, M.D.

My hopes soared.

A couple nights later, as Helmut and I sat entwined in each other's arms on the couch trying to escape in front of the television, the telephone rang, startling the both of us. It was so rare that anyone ever called in the evening – unless the call was from America. I tore myself away from the deeply settled warmth that had developed during the last hour or so of our snuggling hip to hip.

"Hello?"

"Yes, hello," a voice said. "May I speak with Tracie Mayer?"

"Yes, this is she speaking," I said.

"This is Dr. Castañeda calling from Boston."

There was a stunned silence as I felt my skin pimpling into gooseflesh.

"Dr. C...Castañeda?" I glanced at the receiver. Had I heard correctly?

"Dr. Castañeda? I'm sorry," I said, "but this has taken me quite by surprise! This is the Dr. Castañeda, the heart surgeon from Boston, the one I wrote a letter to, that I'm speaking with, right now?"

Helmut clicked the remote control, the picture screen went blank and he turned around towards me, his face one big question mark.

"Yes, this is Dr. Castañeda, and I am in receipt of your letter and that's why I'm calling. How are you?"

"Well, I'm fine, well, I'm not fine, Dr. Castañeda, as you can see by my letter that it may be getting time to do another surgery on our son and the doctors here don't really know what kind of surgery they want to do and me and my husband don't know what to do and I'm beginning to feel like the clock is starting to tick and, Dr. Castañeda, do you know what causes this kind of heart defect?"

"No, Mrs. Mayer –"

"Oh. Tracie, please, call me Tracie, please."

"Okay, Tracie, I'm afraid that we don't know exactly what causes this illness, but we do know that it happens in the very beginning weeks of the pregnancy. Something happens that causes a malformation in the constellation."

"Have you seen this often, Doctor?"

"Well, I have seen variations of course, but the answer is yes."

"Do you think that you could help our son?"

"I'll need some information, but yes, I do think we might be able to help him."

I couldn't believe my ears! I fought to keep the trembling out of my voice – was I dreaming?

I profusely thanked him and replaced the receiver. I looked at Helmut, pointed at the phone and mouthed "THAT WAS DOCTOR CASTAÑEDA!" I jumped up and punched both fists in the air.

"YAHOO! He's seen this kind of disease before and thinks maybe he can help us – I've got to call the University Clinic first thing in the morning so they can get some information ready for me to send to him," I said ripping the top sheet away from the notepad where I'd been jotting down the particulars of the information Doctor Castañeda requested. "I can't believe it! I just can't believe it! Tell me 'Wait till we open him up' my ass!"

Helmut rose from the couch. "Sweetie, wait! – Slow down – tell me what—"

"Can you even believe he called? Helmut! And without even a secretary to make the connection – he himself was on the phone! He asked to speak to me! Doctors don't do that! Hah!

"OhmyGodohmyGodOHMYGOD! Helmut! I didn't even have the street address from the hospital – I just put the name of the hospital, his name and Boston—"

"What just happened?"

"—with the zip code on the envelope! Can you believe it! With all the people this man has to deal with – he takes the time to personally call us! I can't stand it! I didn't even tell you! While you were in Hannover I was sitting in the store reading my magazine – let me get the little booklet and I'll show you where I found him! HALLELUJAH!" I jumped in the air and did a little jig.

Helmut was grinning ear to ear. At the time, I didn't know that this was the same surgeon in Boston my mother had reached out to before Marc's first surgery. The same surgeon who had called the University Clinic while the Professor was away at a seminar and asked the doctors to perform some kind of surgery to bide time. The same surgeon those doctors mimicked. I flew back down the stairs to the kitchen with the booklet and the copy of the letters I had sent, out of breath and beside myself.

I tried to calm down and explain everything. And then I said it all again because the words just felt so good and rang so nicely in my ears and I just wanted to wallow and roll in the sensation of finally, finally being taken by the hand. I had hope enough and to spare.

But suddenly, I was seized with that wretched urge to double-check. The realization struck me that I had to find someone who could tell me something more about one of America's best doctors who just personally called me offering hope of Nirvana. This was demented, I know, but I needed to be sure. Now.

It was ten thirty at night. He would surely be awake. If he wasn't, well, I'd just have to apologize, but he was gonna have to wake up.

The telephone rang twice. "Hello?"

"Dr. Gillor? Hi, it's me, Tracie. HowareyoudidIwakeyouuup?"

"Hello, Tracie. I'm doing well, thank you, especially now that you call me at such a wonderful time."

"Oh, Dr. Gillor – I feel awful calling you so late but you know I wouldn't call if it wasn't really important."

"You didn't wake me, you know I'm only kidding you," he said. "Tell me, what can I do for you?" Dr. Gillor had always been there for me.

Sometime during the past few years, he had left the University Clinic and was now director of the Children's Department of Cardiology at Children's Hospital in Cologne. In the near future, he would be Marc's primary children's cardiologist. I explained everything to him.

"He just called you?" he said.

"Yes! I just hung up the phone with him right now. Do you know him?"

"Well, yes, of course I know him."

"So what do you know about him? Um-hm. Um-hm...okay...and so what kind of surgeon is he – I mean, would you let him operate on your child?...Really! Um-hm. Got it!"

"What's he saying?" Helmut said. I tapped the air in his direction with my index finger signaling him to be quiet and wait a minute.

"...and you're sure," I said finally.

Poor Helmut. He was ready to pop. In my haste, I didn't think to put the loud speaker on. But neither did he. I slowly hung up the phone.

"So Helmut, Dr. Gillor said that he knows of Dr. Castañeda and that he's even attended his seminars when he was here in Germany, and that Dr. Castañeda really is quite famous. And yes, he said he would let him operate on his child and then –" I stepped closer to Helmut so that we stood toe to toe. Cupping his face into my hands, I stared into his eyes. I started off in a whisper.

"He said, 'So, Tracie, let me put it to you like this: You have surgeons and then you have very good surgeons and then you have very, very good surgeons...AND THEN YOU HAVE DR. CASTAÑEDA!!!'"

CHAPTER TWENTY-SEVEN

Shame on You

Hello Dr. Castaneda,
    Greetings from Germany. I really have to take a moment here and thank you once again for your call. You really have no idea how totally surprised I was (and unprepared). I cannot express my appreciation.

Dr. Castaneda; I am sending you here the translated reports from Marc's catheterization of 1991 and his checkup from January of this year. Again, this information is limited; however I would like to know your opinion of these findings. I shall phone you next week and perhaps your secretary can tell me a convenient time to reach you.

I hope this fax finds you well, Dr. Castaneda, have a nice day and again

Thank you very much,
Tracie, February 11, 1994

February 14, Dr. Castañeda phoned again. He wanted to see the last catheter film itself.

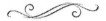

February 17, I greeted the Federal Express driver delivery person at our front door. I said a silent prayer for its safekeeping as he took the package from my hands. I watched him turn, walk down the steps, climb up into his truck, fumble with something for a moment and then watched him back slowly out of our driveway. He glanced up to see me still staring at him. He waved as he put the van in first gear and drove away.

I called Boston the following day. I found out that the package was delivered on February 18, into the hands of a Mr. T. Smith in receiving at 10:36 that morning who forwarded it to the mailroom whereupon it came into the hands of a Ms. S. Perkins from Dr. Mayer's office who delivered it to a Ms. K. Milligan, the manager of cardiac surgery who would personally give it to Dr. Castañeda.

Hello Dr. Castañeda,
Attached please find the following reports:
March 1985 – after Marc's first surgery,
December 1985 – after Marc's second surgery,
August 1991 – his catheterization and
Jan. 1994 – Marc's most recent checkup.

Thank you once again for your attention in my son's case.
Sincerely,
Tracie

April 2, 1994, I received the following fax:

Dear Mrs. Frank-Mayer:
I reviewed the latest cineangiogram and also the cardiac catheterization data and, although your son certainly has a very complex problem, I do think that there is a chance to improve him significantly. At a repeat catheterization here, one should get into the left pulmonary artery or at least obtain bilateral pulmonary venous wedge pressures. From a surgical point of view, one has to first eliminate both left and right Blalock-Taussig shunts, reconstruct the left and right pulmonary arteries, and also communicate the left and right pulmonary arteries centrally, since there is a severe obstruction between these two vessels. Depending on how much time one has to spend doing that, one can either complete the fenestrated Fontan operation or interpose a bidirectional cavopulmonary shunt followed 8 to 10 months later by the fenestrated Fontan operation and then at the second stage complete the fenestrated modification that we developed here for the Fontan operation. I would not be in favor of a repeat palliative shunt operation on the left side; this would just add to the pathophysiology and anatomic complexity.
I hope this information is of value to you.

Best wishes.
Sincerely yours,
Aldo R. Castaneda, M.D.

The following day, Easter Sunday, we three set off in the car headed towards France for a week. This was the first journey, the first time ever in fact, that Helmut and I ever experienced a tentative sense of repose and dared to sit back and embrace a respite away from the edge of the anxious seat. We were reduced to silent smiles as Marc quietly sang in the backseat while outside the countryside rolled by and the sheep grazed and every now and again a village cloistered around its church steeple and the flowers grew wild and everything seemed right. Finally. It was, indeed, the first time in our lives as parents that anyone had ever given us hope for our son.

Ever.

The Monday morning following our Sunday night return, Marc stayed home from school with a fever, vomiting and diarrhea. Helmut went to work. I called Lufthansa Airlines and instructed them to pull our files – if they in fact still existed – and prepare the necessary documentation we would need for our flight to Boston.

Then I called the University Clinic for the first available appointment with the Professor.

"Good afternoon, Children's Cardiology Department. You're speaking with Nurse Barbara."

"*Guten Tag* Nurse Barbara. Tracie Mayer here. *Ich Grüsse Sie.*" ("I greet you.")

"*Guten Tag* Frau Mayer, I greet you too."

"Does the Professor have a moment to see me today?"

"Is Marc not well?" she asked me.

"Marc is okay. It's me. I must see the Professor as soon as possible. It's urgent." I told her.

"Let me see...Frau Mayer, can you come by late this afternoon, say between five and six o'clock?"

That would be perfect – by then Helmut would have received the faxed information from the airlines which I could stop by and pick up on my way. If it was the same document as the one before, the Professor would need all of a minute to fill it out and sign it. I remember thinking that he would feel better – not even better – he'd feel great about filling it out this time around and sign it in a jiffy, happy and relieved at our good fortune.

"That'll be fine!" I said. "I'll be there," trailed the receiver as I hung up the phone in a rush.

The fax from the airlines, which indeed turned out to be the same document as the previous one when we flew to America five years before, lay on the seat next to me, inserted in transparent plastic, safe and secure out of the smudge and crumple zone. I was all torn up inside. Mustered up every ounce of courage I had. Prayed for vision. Forced myself to slow down at the yellow lights. Were we doing the right thing? It was five minutes before midnight – what were our options? Couldn't stay here. Dr. Castañeda was offering us hope and a plan to save Marc. Here, the doctors didn't know what to do.

You know this is really a no-brainer, I told myself. It's just that I'm used to the doctors here. "Have you lost your last goddamn mind? Somethin' beats the hell out of nothin' all day long. Don't go stupid on me now. You know your daddy didn't raise no dummies!" Daddy's voice rang in my ears. Had to maintain a brave face for Helmut. A big, big chill was swelling around his feet: "What if these Americans don't really know what they're doing?" he was starting to wonder too often aloud.

"They know what they're doing, they know what they're doing, don't be afraid, ol' girl," I told myself. "After all, the third time's the charm. Best things come in threes, and if you don't believe these old wives' tales then you'd better believe in your family unit which is you and Marc and Helmut, one, two, three and that it's going to remain that way. Believe it! Have to let Marc's teacher know...on second thought, maybe not. She'd probably mean well, but I could just see her standing at the head of the classroom, calling her students to attention and then sharing with them the fact that 'MARC MAYER IS GOING TO AMERICA TO GO TO THE HOSPITAL AND HAVE HEART SURGERY AND

MARC WE WILL BE THINKING ABOUT YOU...ARE YOU AFRAID?'

"No, no. I've got to downplay this as much as possible. Marc's got to have a most positive mind-set. There's something in Proverbs...what is it? Oh, yes. A merry heart is as good as medicine. That's right, that's it, I don't doubt that at all. Take it all one minute at a time and keep your eye on your goal. Can't allow Marc for one minute to be unduly frightened. Got to go into this thing with the right spirit.

"I know what I'll do – I'll tell the school director instead. Yep, that's what I'll do and I'll do it the day before we go. That way, there's no chance of Marc having to deal with this with his classmates. And I'll just tell him – what's the guy's name? Doesn't matter, that we would appreciate it greatly if when he shared this information with the teacher that he be kind enough to ask her to keep her mouth shut about it.

"I have to pack. I wonder what the temperature is there now – not that it really matters anyway, but I'll just ask somebody in Boston the next time I speak to them which will probably be tonight. Man! If everything could be so easy. I'll call the German Rescue Squad when I – well, maybe I won't have to call because maybe we won't even need a doctor to take with us. We ended up not needing one the last time. Yeah, but the last time Marc wasn't about to face surgery either. Okay, don't fret, don't fret. Let's just wait and see what the Professor thinks is the best thing to do.

"I wonder if Helmut reached Cheryl about the insurance. Hope Marc's bug is gone before we go...Lord, we are about to make a decision that will affect the rest of our lives. Please help Helmut and me to see clearly through our tension. Help me to bury my anxiety. Reassure me. And please, please for our child's sake, let us be doing the right thing."

The gate was up. I drove into the grounds. Like all mothers, I believed God would make everything all right.

In about eight minutes I would be thunderstruck.

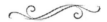

"Maybe you didn't understand me Professor," I said.

Each of us examined the other as I rose, slowly circled my chair, stationed myself behind it and with outstretched arms leaned onto its top splat. My eyes bored into his.

"So I'm going to repeat myself. Dr. Castañeda, whom you know, is preparing to do surgery on Marc immediately. He has told me personally over the telephone that he and his team have an operation that will significantly – understand me correctly – significantly improve Marc's health. Helmut and I are, as you and I speak Professor, making arrangements with the hospital, the hotel and the airlines. Now all I need you to do is fill out that paper there for Lufthansa."

"Frau—"

"What Professor? It's the same document as the one you filled out the last time we flew to America and I don't understand why we are even having this conversation. Just please fill it out and sign it!"

"Frau Mayer, I really don't see this as necessary."

The knot knotting in my chest was about to asphyxiate me.

"What do you mean you don't see it as necessary? You know better than anyone else that if Marc needs oxygen during the flight, the airlines have to be notified beforehand! You're the one who scared the daylights out of me the last time we flew – What did you say? As I recall it was something like, 'It's not a good idea – the authorities would have to be informed – IS IT REALLY NECESSARY?' Well Professor – this is necessary. This trip is really, really necessary. This trip is so necessary I can BARELY SEE STRAIGHT!"

"Frau Mayer," he said, looking at the document, "I cannot si –"

"Wait a minute! Wait...just...one...minute," I said slicing my hand through the air the way Uncle Boo always did when he didn't want to hear anymore. The conversation was beginning to stagger my mind. A shake of my head stressed my disbelief.

"Professor, with all due respect, you still don't seem to get it. We don't have time for what you cannot do!" I said walking over to his desk and pointing my finger at the document. "I know I'm repeating myself, but you aren't giving me any choice. Again, this-is-the-same-document-you-filled-out-and signed the last time we flew to America! So why won't you sign this one? Where is the issue here? If it's a matter of time – and I know it will only take all of three minutes – I am prepared to wait!"

"I don't see any necessity for him to go to Boston," he said.

Whoa Nelly.

"You, you what? YOU WHAT? What do you mean you don't see the necessity of him going to Boston?"

"Frau Mayer," he said. "If I sign this paper for you to take him to America, it would be like an admission that our surgeons here are not qualified to operate on him and—"

"WELL, THEY'RE NOT!" I backed away from him and began to pace the room, counting out the critical issues on my hand.

"Now – let me get this straight: are you telling me that I had the absolute fortune of making contact with one of the leading heart surgeons in the world who understands the urgency of our situation, who knows what procedure he plans to perform to save my child's life and is preparing his team and on top of all this – is the only person on this planet to ever have given me and Helmut any hope about Marc's future and we should not go running to him? Are you serious? I mean, do you really expect me to let you people operate on him and you don't even know what you intend to do? Is that what you are trying to tell me? Tell me that I've got it all wrong, Professor, tell me—"

"Frau Mayer, I must support my surgeons."

I eased myself once again onto the edge of my chair. Caught my breath. A long measured moment hung in the air before I spoke. Should I come at him from a position of strength? Should I beg? You know, I've never really been a damsel in distress type of girl, but at that particular moment, I thought I would succumb. 'You'll get more flies with sugar than with shit, sweetheart.'

'Bullshit Theresa! Don't tell our child that! You listen to your daddy and stay on his ass, Tracie! You know it ain't no givin' up and no givin' out! Tell that man to sign the goddamn paper or you'll have pickets in front of the hospital and in front of his house at nine o'clock sharp in the morning!' I leaned forward, propped my elbows on his desk and rested my chin on the back of my hands. Looked him square in the eye. Considering my predicament, when I first spoke, it seemed as if I'd been dusted with a hypnotic calm.

"What would you...choose for your child, Professor?"

"Frau Mayer—"

"WHAT WOULD YOU CHOOSE FOR YOUR CHILD, PROFESSOR?" I leaped out of my chair knocking it over. "THIS IS MY CHILD'S LIFE WE'RE TALKING ABOUT HERE GODDAMNIT! How dare you be more concerned with what someone will think about what your surgeons are doing than what you can to help me save this child's life! Forget being a doctor for a minute!" I said with a thwack of my open palm on his desk. "Where is your sense of compassion for Christ's sake?"

He stared at the document while fiddling self-consciously with it as if his fingers were stuck not only to its transparent packaging, but to the right and wrong and life and death of the situation. The hovering silence swelled to a crescendo, then burst like a bomb all around me. My flare-up had made no impact. Apparently that gray matter of his brain controlling his comprehension as well as the factor affecting his emotion had shut down.

"I can't sign it," he said.

He wouldn't look at me. I walked over and snatched the cellophane out of his hand and rested my knuckles on his desk. I stood there, looming over him, inches away from his face, blinded by fury and probably frothing at the mouth but I refused to let the tears fall.

"Let me tell you something," I said. "I've been going through hell for nine years – NINE YEARS! And you know what they say? They say that if you're going through hell just keep on going through it because you will eventually come out on the other side and THAT is JUST what I intend do with or without your help.

"And-believe-you-me one more thing: not you, not your surgeons, not NOBODY – NOT NO GODDAMN BODY IS GOING TO GET IN THE WAY OF ME SAVING MY CHILD'S LIFE! YOU GOT THAT? NOBODY! And you must be insane if you think otherwise." I walked to the door, and yanked it open.

"Shame on you," I said.

Later that evening Helmut called him at home. He needn't have bothered.

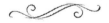

The following week went by in a flurry. Everything came to a head on April 19th. That morning, I called Dr. Tinschman. He told me that he would fill out the documents for me. I needed to stop by his office anyway so he could listen to Marc's lungs and see how he was faring. And true to his word, he filled out the document. It read in part:

EDA 04: Prognosis for the trip? No problem expected, (the child) has flown several times.

EDA 09: Shall passenger be escorted: For any cardiac incidents, a doctor to escort the child would be recommended.

I faxed the paper back to Lufthansa at noon. By five thirty that early evening I would have eaten shit with the buzzards for just a scintilla of serenity. By eight thirty that night, I was ready to blow my brains out.

Upon receiving the fax, Lufthansa once again rejected our request because the document again was not signed by the Professor and before the German Rescue Squad could decide who and under what conditions someone would accompany us to Boston, they would need that information from Lufthansa which Lufthansa of course could not give them, and since that was the case, the Rescue Squad would need to talk to the cardiologist, so of course to cut to the quick of the matter, I called Dr. Castañeda who was in surgery, but thankfully Dr. Freed, his cardiologist colleague was available and he told me that he didn't believe Marc needed any assistance, and that even if he did, it would only likely be minimal and if that were to happen, the airlines have emergency oxygen on board.

He was sure Marc could make it, but he would definitely speak with the German Rescue Squad if that would give me peace of mind.

So in between trying to beat the clock with the six-hour time difference and busy signals in order to hook up this one to speak with that one and getting the final cost breakdown from Miss Coulomb in Boston on the hospital expense for Herr Götzle representing the insurance company in Germany, which for the past couple days had been trying to understand why the operation had to be carried out in America anyway, and making room reservations for Soon, Real Soon, This Month 1994, and worrying about who was going to take care of our dog, and swallowing my heart back down to where it belonged yet continuing to smile while observing Marc sit on the floor and tap the ping-pong ball against the paddle three times before tiring and me saying, "It's okay, little man, we're getting ready to go see Dr. Castañeda and he's going to make you feel so much better and you're not going to be out of breath anymore," and in the next moment sounding completely addle-headed speaking on the phone with our internist (who was now returning my call at the end of his busy day) as I tried to remember just why I had placed a call to him earlier (which was to find out Helmut's and my blood groups), I pleaded our case again that evening with Lufthansa whose Frau Sommer informed me that now under no uncertain terms could we fly with them.

Someone from the Professor's office had warned them about Marc's condition and they were not willing to take the chance and let us fly with them.

"I'm sorry," she said.

CHAPTER TWENTY-EIGHT

Sky High

Maybe there's something to that saying that there's only so much crap in life you have to eat because when we flew to Boston exactly one week later, there was: no doctor from the German Rescue Squad to accompany us, no medical document from Lufthansa, no Lufthansa, no mention of Marc's health prior to take off, while airborne, nor at touchdown, and though there was no cessation of my dry heaves during the flight...there was no problem in the sky.

CHAPTER TWENTY-NINE

Children's Boston

My bottom lip dropped when the doors slid open smooth as water to a larger than life-sized carousel horse – hanging suspended from the ceiling. Walls drifted in and out of varying shades of green while others blushed fuchsia by degrees. A tightly woven textured carpet hugged the floor all over, muffling all click-clacks, taps and squeaks. A sign posted near a looking glass elevator announced the upcoming entertainment to be performed a few steps away in the auditorium on a stage presently hidden from view courtesy of velvet rippling scarlet curtains.

Not wanting to miss a thing, I deliberately turned around ever so slowly and the first glimpse of a beautiful Wurlitzer jukebox stopped me in my tracks and then lured me to its side to stroke its shiny mahogany – and suddenly Marc shrieked. My head snapped in his direction. His eyes bulged out of their sockets. His mouth looked ready to shout hosannas. He clapped his hands and then rubbed them together as he tentatively approached it in disbelief. Helmut looked up from the thick of the action in a corner of activity. There was no one else around. Marc stepped closer and closer until he could just have at it. Lo and behold, the most wondrous of wonders for a nine-year-old boy: an arcade- sized Nintendo! "So this is Boston Children's Hospital," I said to myself smiling.

After our check-in at the hospital, we went directly to the hotel, The Children's Inn, which was, just as we'd been told, built directly adjacent to the hospital. It had been constructed with the specific purpose of housing the parents and family members of the hospital patients.

"Welcome to our hotel," the young woman behind the counter said.

"Oh, thank you," I said. "We are the Mayers from Germany."

"Oh, Mrs. Mayer! You made it! We're so happy you're here. Did you have a nice flight? That's a pretty long way away! My name's Regina," she said extending her hand towards me, smiling.

"Yes, it was fine," I said, pumping her hand, so happy, happy, happy to be grinding my soles onto terra firma.

She smiled at Helmut. "Welcome Mr. Mayer," she said.

"*Hallo*," he said. "Thank you."

She leaned over the counter towards Marc. "Hi! You must be Marc. I'll bet you must be pooped after such a long trip!"

"*Hallo*," Marc said briefly smiling and then looking quickly up to Helmut and whispering, "*Papa, was ist pooped?*" ("What is pooped?")

"Weiß ich auch nicht," Helmut said. ("I don't know either.")

"It means tired, sweetie," I said looking down at Marc, stroking the back of his head.

Regina looked at us and smiled in between shuffling a few papers.

"Listen," she said. "I'm going to need just a moment of your time to fill out these papers – Mrs. Mayer, do you want to have the honors?"

"Sure," I said. Helmut nodded in agreement.

"Mr. Mayer, would you and Marc like to go up to your room and get settled while your wife fills out the papers? It won't take long."

"Yes, that would be good," he said. She handed Marc the key.

"Come with me, Marc. Let's go upstairs to the room and wait for Mama. She has to fill out some papers and that will take a few minutes."

"I'll be there soon," I said over my shoulder as they walked towards the elevator.

"So," I said turning back to the clerk, rat-a-tat-tatting my nails against the counter. "What papers do you have for me to fill out?"

She placed her cool hand over my clammy one. The moment was almost too much. If it was her empathy or my angst or just hearing my language floating all about me, or all of the above – it was just too much. My eyes began to fill. I couldn't help it.

"Listen," she said leaning intimately over the counter towards me. "Don't worry. Everything will be fine. Do you mind me asking what your handsome little boy is here for? It's okay if you don't w–"

"He's here for heart surgery," I said. "This will be the third time. The first two were done in Germany where we live."

"Well, you can be rest assured," she said, "that he is really in good hands. This is a great hospital," she said squeezing my hand briefly before pulling away.

"We're – he's going to be operated on by Dr. Castañeda," I said.

"Dr. Castañeda!" she said. "Oh I am so happy for you! Wait until you meet him! He is just the nicest man! Hey – Sherry! Come here a minute and tell Mrs. Mayer about Dr. Cas—"

"–taneda?" Sherry said, hanging up the telephone receiver and heading towards us. "So where shall I start? I could literally go on for days." She folded one hand over the other, rested them on the counter separating us, and looked me square in the eye. "He is without question, not only a great surgeon, but I swear, probably just about the nicest, kindest person you'll ever have the chance to meet, right, Dan?"

Dan had just emerged through a door landing him right next to his colleagues.

"Right Dan, what?" he said smiling at me.

"Sherry and I were just telling Mrs. Mayer here about Dr. Castañeda."

He broke out into a big smile and affirmed the consensus with a knowing nod. "Ahh, Dr. Castaneda. We all have him up there around the Big Man himself," he said. "Really a gentleman, one of the nicest people you're likely to meet. And he's a well-respected surgeon, one of the best – if not the best."

"You know, that's the impression I had of him over the telephone," I said. "I mean, not of course about his surgical skills, but his kindness."

"Just wait till you meet him," Dan said.

"See? We weren't exaggerating," Regina said. "And," she went on, "he's got the most beautiful blue eyes!"

"Glad you said it!" Sherry said.

"Okay girls, down, down," Dan said. Laughter erupted all around diminishing some of the sting in my eyes.

"I needed that laugh," I said smiling into each of their faces. "You all have certainly made me feel better. Thank you so much. I really mean it."

I finished filling out the forms and headed for the elevator. The door opened and closed silently behind me. My child's life would soon be in his hands. I let my head rest against the wall, closed my eyes and tried to envision this man called Dr. Castañeda.

CHAPTER THIRTY

Aladdin

After unpacking our suitcases, we headed back towards the hospital. Tacos and cokes were the order of the day as we seated ourselves at one of the blue mesh iron tables on the expansive patio off the cafeteria, squinting our eyes from a sun that shone upon blossoms embroidering a fine green linen of a lawn shimmering in the daylight. Marc wanted to get back to Nintendo. Nothing doing. One thing after the other. Now was time to eat: chew, swallow and build up our strength...our strength.

"I haven't had a taco in years," I said to myself. "I love tacos!"

"Then show a little enthusiasm, will you? You can't gag and pick over this meal and expect Marc to eat and enjoy it, now, can you?" I said.

"'Don't do as I do, do as I say do' won't work here, will it?"

"No."

I felt like eating that taco, or anything else for that matter, about as much as I felt like having a hole drilled into my head.

Nonetheless, I sunk my teeth into a crunchy, spicy, meaty, lettucy bite.

"Umm. Tastes good!" I said looking to Marc and Helmut.

"Does it taste good to you both too?" They chewed and nodded in agreement.

My senses picked up the soft sound of water streaming steadily, indeed resolutely, in a fountain that soared from the center of the tended grounds:

unafraid,

undaunted,

unshakable.

The echocardiogram would begin at three thirty.

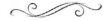

The young woman commissioned to the charge of performing the echogram invited us into the room with a welcoming gesture. Her winning personality put me at ease immediately. She guided Marc towards the exam bed.

"So, you're Marc! It's nice to meet you. You're pretty big for nine!" she said.

Marc smiled. "Nice to meet you too," he said extending his hand.

"So now, before we get down to business, young man, I have just one question."

Marc had lain down, his fingers laced behind his head. He looked up at her.

"*Nämlich?*" he said. ("That is?")

"You have to speak English with her Mouse," I said.

"Oh, *ja*, Mama, I forgot," he said giggling. He looked back at her. "What is your question?" he said.

She stood there, hands on her hips, head cocked to one side. "I was just wondering what your favorite movie is these days," she said.

She didn't have to ask twice. "*Aladdin!*" he said pronouncing it the way that was familiar to him: *Al-la-deen*.

She looked to me for the Americanized translation. "Aha! *Aladdin*...Hmm...Let me see what I can..." She turned on her heels and headed for a cabinet on the other side of the room. A moment later she was back at Marc's side. "Could this be the *Al-la-deen* you're talking about?" she said waving the video before him.

"*Ja!* That's it! That's it! Woo-hoo!" he shouted nearly rolling from the bed with glee. She popped it into the video recorder and Marc's eyes became transfixed to the television screen. This would be the umpteenth time he'd seen this tale unfold, the first time in English. And as soon as it started he was miles away. After a moment, only the animated voices enlivened the muted room. The echocardiogram was underway.

After a time, Helmut motioned me a few feet away from the exam bed.

"Do you really think she knows what she's doing?" he said. "I mean, in Germany, the Professor always made this test." He shook his weary head. "*Ich weiss es nicht ab die Amerikaner wissen was die tun.*" ("I don't know if the Americans know what they are doing.")

"Helmut, look—"

"Don't you think she looks a little young?" he said.

"Helmut, believe me," I said, urging my own self to believe in what I was about to say. "They wouldn't have her here doing this if they thought she wasn't capable of…."

He walked away from me headed in her direction.

"…doing it."

"Excuse me," he said. "Sorry to bother you now, but I'm just wondering how long you do this."

"Oh, probably about the time it takes for Marc to watch the film," she said not moving her eyes from the screen before her.

"No, no, that's not what I mean. I mean, how long, how many years you have been doing this because in Germany, it is the Professor, the leader of the *Kinder Kardiologie Abteilung*" – he looked to me.

"Children's Cardiology Department," I interjected.

"Yes, Children's Cardiology Department – the Professor is the one who always did this exam on Marc."

She smiled at her screen. "Mr. Mayer," she said, "I have been trained to specifically do this kind of work. I'm a specialist with this machine, but I really want you to relax, and I think it would help if you took a peek inside that door over there."

"In that door, over there?" he said pointing to the door we entered.

"No, no. That one," she said. "Over there."

"Aha! Over there," he said.

"Um-hmm," she said without looking up.

Helmut and I kind of tiptoed our way across the room and quietly opened the door. The room was dimly lit. Six doctors sat in silence before their own screens. "They're all watching what I'm doing," she said. Helmut and I looked at each other in amazement.

By the time the last reel of *Al-la-deen* rolled, Marc was standing and buttoning his shirt.

"Wow, Papa! Der Film ist super! Ich habe alles verstanden!" ("Man, Papa! The film is great! I understood everything!") He was beaming.

I stared at my child and silently thanked God for this wonderful day, wondering what tomorrow might bring.

CHAPTER THIRTY-ONE

Paradise

The Second Day. Rolling over onto my side, it felt groggily like morning. Instantly an electrifying sense of awareness sprang up from the bowels of my inertia and jolted me into a blinking awareness. Reality smacked me in the face; I shot up out of the bed and stumbled. My eyes whisked around the room in the waning darkness, my hands groped for familiar. A moment passed before I got my bearings. Cautiously, I sat back down. Wasn't I just sitting here, like this? Damn! This was not my plan.

Several hours before, washed and creamed and pajamaed, I was indeed sitting here on the edge of this queen-sized bed, my back to Helmut. His eyes were closed, but I knew he was not quite sleeping; therefore I had to be very quiet as I went about my business. He hated it when I took any kind of pills. "Well, far be it from me to pooh-pooh his opinion because under normal circumstances, he very well might be right," I remember thinking, rising from my knees after trying to calm myself with a heart-to-heart with God. "Maybe we do get enough vitamins from our food, but that's no consolation for me at this particular point in time, because whenever the thought of eating even crosses my mind lately, my stomach lurches."

"Don't worry about it, girlfriend. This too shall pass. Just keep taking your vitamins."

"You've got that right. I intend to continue taking my vitamins and with the greatest of ease I am going to slip this sweet little sleeping pill here underneath my tongue, and pay special attention to how it slowly dissolves."

I peeled the crisp white sheet and the blanket back, slid in, reached up to switch off the night lamp, scooted down into the cool freshness of the bedclothes, pulled them up underneath my armpits and gently rested my head on the pillow.

"And I don't want to be lulled, I don't want to be lullabied, my only desire is to really, really enjoy the disintegration of this pill and hail the moment when I know I'm about to drift off and sleep the sleep of the just without a guilty conscience because right now, at this very moment Marc is fine, he is comfortable, his room is wonderful, the nurses are attentive and reassuring and there's a call button right next to him if he needs anything and Dr. Castañeda is never too far away.

"Yes, I will relish this moment and I will recognize that I am relishing this moment and how good it really feels. And I will be thankful..." I nuzzled further down into the covers. "This kind of feels like what a thick juicy bacon avocado cheeseburger tastes like on a good day. I swear if everything continues this smoothly I will consider us to be so very blessed. Just think. Twenty-four hours ago we had no idea what was in store for us and up until now, everything's turned out to be better than what we could ever have even imagined. And good Lord am I thankful that Helmut is pleased! If he peered at me one more time with his skeptical eyes I don't know what I was going to do...Whew."

Tossing, turning, urging my little helper to produce its desired effects, the events of the day continued to scroll beneath my curtained eyes.

"Six East. That's where Marc's room is."

"Don't think! You're just going to keep yourself wound up and just when you start to fall off, it'll be time to get up and function."

"I'm trying! Maybe once I play everything through, I'll be able to relax. Now just leave me alone while I do this! So let's see...Which route did we take from the echo lab to Marc's room? I can't remember, but it was a pretty good trek. Maybe it seems longer because we kept at Marc's pace. I do remember standing there as the door was opened, looking around and thinking: Wow! If Daddy could see this place he'd try to get at least six-fifty for it. And then as if on cue, Marc and Helmut and I all stepped inside and set off in different directions. The woman who ushered us in accompanied us inside and pointed out some details about the room. First, she walked over to Marc's bed, sat down and patted the empty space alongside her.

"My name's Maureen," she said looking towards Marc. Marc accepted her invitation and told her his name.

"Nice to meet you," she said shaking his hand.

"*Nett Dich auch kennen zu lernen,* um, I mean, nice to meet you too," he said.

"Hey, buddy, you're doing a great job with all that English and German. Maybe you can teach me a few words before you go home."

"Okay," Marc said. "*Warum nicht?*"

"Okay, help me out here. What did you just say?"

"Why not?" Marc smiled up at her.

"Waru – say it again," she said.

Marc repeated it and she did the same.

"Yes, you see? German is not so difficult – just ask my mom."

I rolled my eyes up to the ceiling and everybody laughed.

"Well, since you've given me my first German lesson," Maureen said, "I think it's only fair that I give you some information." She turned the television on as she continued. "I think you'll be pleased to know that the television here has about eighteen channels, a few your mom and dad might like to watch too," she said throwing a wink my way. "And there's one really special program you'll find on channel 22. This is Children's in-house TV channel. Here you can watch movies from nine in the morning 'til eleven at night —"

"Wow!" Marc said.

"But I'm sure you won't want to watch television so late, will you?" she said.

He looked up at her and laughed. "That's what I thought," she said. "And, on Tuesdays, the Patient Entertainment Center, did you see the room near the jukebox with the red curtains when you first got here?"

"Yes," Marc said wide eyed.

"Well that room is what we call the Patient Entertainment Center – PEC for short, anyhow, on Tuesdays, the PEC becomes a television studio with lights, cameras and lots of action. And you can go down and be a part of the show or enjoy it right here in your room. And in the evenings you can go down there and there'll be some kind of fun stuff going on—"

"Yeah?" Marc said.

"Um-hmm," she said

"Like what?" Marc said.

"Oh, like magic shows and clowns and storytellers. It's a lot of fun."

"Hey, *euch beiden*," he said shooting smiling eyes over to Helmut and me, "*das ist gar nicht so schlecht!*" ("Hey, you two, this isn't so bad!")

"*Marc, das ist super!*" Helmut said.

"You should tell Maureen that, Marc," I said.

"This is pretty good, here," Marc said grinning up at her.

"Thought you might like that. Why don't you kick your shoes off and stay a while? Here's the remote control," she said as she handed it to him. She then rose from the bed and walked towards me.

"Thanks," Marc said kicking his shoes off and curling himself up on top of the bed.

"I'm Maureen Sullivan," she said extending her hand. "I'm your Patient Care Coordinator."

"Hi, I'm Tracie Mayer."

"Welcome to Children's," she said.

"Thank you."

290 · TRACIE FRANK MAYER

"So will either you or Mr. Mayer be rooming in?"

"No, we've checked into The Inn next door."

"Okay, that's good, you'll have a little more space, but if you should decide to stay, the bathroom is over there –"

"Oh good, excuse me," Helmut said and disappeared inside.

"And this couch over here converts to a bed, there's a locker over there by Marc's bed and if you should decide to stay, let me know and if you need one, I can get you a 'Parent Pack' which has a blanket, couple of sheets, towels, a pillow and facecloth."

"Okay, thank you very much," I said.

"Everything else you may need to know about Children's is in the info packet for you there on the table. Read through it and if you have any questions, feel free to ask me or any of the attending nurses. I'll be back around later this evening."

Helmut stepped out of the bathroom. "Mr. Mayer, I hope you enjoy your stay," she said heading out the door.

"Oh! Thank you," he said.

"Thank you, Mrs. or is it Ms. Sullivan?" I said.

"It's Mrs., but please call me Maureen."

"Okay, if you'll call me Tracie."

She smiled. "Okay, Tracie, see you all later," and she closed the door quietly behind her.

"What a nice lady, you guys, huh?"

"Maybe she's nice, but what did she mean? I'm not here for a vacation, how shall I enjoy my stay?"

"Oh, Helmut – you know what she meant."

"*Ja, ja.* I know. It was just a joke. Sweetie, come look at the bathroom. It's so big! It's really nice. And the soap smells real good."

"It must. I can see you've scrubbed your face. I hope you didn't dirty any of the towels – they're for Marc," I said sitting down on the couch with the information pack.

"Mama! Papa! Look!" Marc said, his eyes riveted on the television.

"What, my son?" Helmut said heading over towards the window. Marc didn't look away from the screen. Suddenly he cracked up laughing at the cartoon voices. After a moment, he became quiet and looked over at me with raised eyebrows as if to say: look what I've got for you! as da da da dadadadaa da filled the void in the air and then a news reporter said, "Welcome back. You're watching CNN and these are the headlines at this hour." Then he immediately switched again and it was Elmo. Snoopy. ABC. CBS. Disney. Marc laid propped back on the pillow spellbound as he channel-surfed with the remote control.

"Man, is this a big hospital," Helmut said craning his neck, looking as far as he could see out the window.

"Um-hmm," I said not lifting my eyes from the Contents page of: A Guide for Patients and Parents. He ambled by, looked at me, asked me what I was reading and then sunk himself down onto the couch next to me. After a moment, he shifted abruptly. Twice. Three times.

"Helmut, can you please st – "

"Hey! Look here!" he said continuing to fiddle with something on the side of the couch. "You can push this button here and the couch pulls out to a bed!"

"I know that already."

"Hey, Papa!"

"Marc, honey, can you please turn that down a little bit for Mom? I'm trying to read this important information here."

"Okay, Mom. Papa! There are so many programs just for kids! Look!"

The Chipmunks. Click. Lassie. Click. Three Ninjas.

Click – "*NEIN! DAS GIBTS NICHT! AL-A-DEEN!*" ("NO! THAT'S NOT POSSIBLE! ALADDIN!")

"Marc! Have you lost your mind? Quiet down! You can't shout like that in here!" I said.

Right at that moment, we all fell silent and looked at each other. We thought we heard the tail end of it, but we weren't quite sure, so we ignored what we thought we may have heard until we heard it again a moment later, a bit louder this time – I pounded once against my knee and said, "See? Damn it!" – and we all hesitantly called out "Come in!" and the door opened and there he stood smiling and I knew it was him.

Marc looked over at him and without a word, straightened himself up on the bed and turned the television down. He was not what I expected. But then again, what did I expect? He stood erect. Tall. Slender. Elegant. His head crowned in a cloud of white hair neatly trimmed, parted on the side; thick but tamed snow-white eyebrows capped glass-framed eyes the color of forget-me-nots. In full bloom. He glided over to Marc and extended his hand.

"*Hallo*," he said. "*Ich bin Dr. Castañeda.* "*Du bist bestimmt der Marc.*" ("I am Dr. Castaneda. You must be Marc.")

"*Ja. Ich bin der Marc. Guten Tag.*" ("Yes, I am Marc. Good day.")

"*Guten Tag,*" he said sitting down next to him on the bed.

"*Sprichst Du lieber English oder Deutsch?*" ("Do you prefer to speak English or German?") Dr. Castañeda said.

"*Für mich ist es egal. Die Frage ist, was sprechen Sie lieber?*" ("For me it doesn't matter. The question is what do you prefer to speak?") Marc said.

Dr. Castañeda laughed and then carried on in perfect German.

"Well, my German is probably not as good as yours, but we can speak German with one another if you like."

"Okay, fine, then German," Marc said.

"So tell me. How do you feel?"

"Oh, I'm fine," Marc said.

"I'm happy about that. Have you discovered all the great television programs yet?" Dr. Castañeda said.

"Yes! They're great!"

He ruffled Marc's hair. Marc didn't shy away.

Helmut and I walked over and met him at the foot of Marc's bed.

"Mrs. Mayer," he said taking my hand. "I'm so glad you're here. Welcome, welcome to Boston. Welcome to Children's."

"Dr. Ca–," I nodded and perhaps even curtsied as I tried to clear the lump out of my throat. My eyes swelled and the best I could do was a feeble attempt at a smile.

He patted my arm. "Everything will be fine," he said. And then he looked to Helmut who grasped his hand. He covered Helmut's hand with his other as they shook.

"*Herr Mayer. Herzlich willkommen. Hoffentlich haben Sie eine schöne Reise gehabt.*" ("You are warmly welcomed. Hopefully, you had a nice trip.")

"*Danke, haben wir.*" Helmut said. ("Thank you, we did.")

"And you had no problems?"

"Not at all," Helmut said.

I watched in plain English as it registered on Helmut's face.

"Dr. Castañeda, *Sie sprechen aber perfektes Deutsch! Das ist eine Überraschung!*" Helmut said. ("Dr. Castañeda, you speak perfect German! That is a surprise!")

"Well, yes, I can speak a few words."

"I certainly didn't expect that! Do you have perhaps a moment's time? I have a few questions."

"Of course," Dr. Castañeda said and extended his hand toward the couch. I watched the two of them get seated while I slowly cushioned myself near the foot of Marc's bed and pinched myself.

Shaky!

Speechless!

Splendiferous!

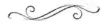

"Boy! What a day...I wonder if Marc is sleeping yet. That Nintendo thing or whatever it was they hooked up to his television earlier will surely entice him to stay awake and play. But the nurses said they'd peek in on him periodically throughout the night. He's such a good kid. He'll get some sleep—"

"You'd better get some sleep, girlie." My alter ego again.

"He knows we have another busy day tomorrow," I went on, ignoring myself. "He doesn't seem to be anxious at all. That's so typical Marc. He has no idea that he is the very conduit through which I receive my strength. I'm so thankful...and I'm so worried, I'm so damn worried and afraid and afraid of being so afraid and—"

"Stop tangling with it! Don't let the demons in! Everything will be fine! Believe it! What does Mama always say? Let go and let God. Do it! I mean it now! Relax... Give your pill the chance... to kick in. Come back...to the burger."

"Okay, okay. You're...right. I'm, I'm fine. It's all good... Everything will be fine. I...I do wonder...what Marc's really thinking, though."

"Tracie, relax now. Think about...it...tomorrow."

"It is ...the strangest sensation doing this...this hospital thing...English. Have to reacquaint myself. How to speak...strangers...in my language...daily basis – but just for a short time, hopefully...did you hear that, God? The part about...about short time?...Glad...laid clothes out already...so tired...want to think...as little as...poss..."

The few hours from then till now had flown by like a shooting star. And now in the half light of daybreak, I felt and no doubt looked as if someone had raised the alarm. Marc was scheduled for a cardiac catheterization today.

"Relax. Lay back down. It's only a quarter to five. That's it. Calm. Everything will be okay."

"I wish I could wake Helmut up to confirm that for me."

"Maybe he is awake."

"Helmut?" I said, barely more than a whisper.

"Hmmm?" he said.

"Are you sleeping?"

He tapped and patted against the sheets until his hand brushed against my face. He tweaked my nose and then rested his hand on my collarbone.

"No, I'm awake. A long time."

I slid over closer to him. His hand shifted, rounding around my shoulder. He gripped me firmly.

"So today they make the catheter," he said.

"Um-hm."

"Okay," he sighed. "Do you know which doctor will do it?"

"No." His hand shifted a bit.

"You know in Germany the Professor always did it."

"I know that, Helmut."

"Do you think we should ask?"

"Do I think we should ask what?"

"Who will make the catheter."

"If you knew the person's name would it make any difference to you? We don't know him or her anyhow, so why should we ask? When the Professor made the first catheter when Marc wasn't even two weeks old, did we know him? No we didn't and—"

"Yes, but I trusted him because I knew that because he was the Professor he was the best."

I inhaled deeply and exhaled through partially opened lips and Dizzy Gillespie cheeks. "Okay. Well, tell me this. How do you feel about things so far?" I said.

"*Gut.*"

"You think we've got Marc in good hands," I said.

"Yes, no question."

"Well, then you certainly don't think that this hospital and Dr. Castañeda for Christ's sake, would have someone stick a long skinny tube into a vein in Marc's groin and snake it all the way up to his heart who was mentally deficient, do you?" I sat up and looked down at him.

"What is def– ?"

"Incompetent! Stupid! *Blöd!* You know what I'm trying to say!"

"Don't start with the damn screaming so early in the morning!"

My head plopped back down onto the pillow. Screaming. I forgot the screaming. He hated pills and screaming. His nerves were bad. My nerves were bad. I wasn't screaming, just trying to make a point that slipped out an octave higher.

We listened to each other breathe for a moment. After a time he said, "What has to be, has to be. Shit."

He rolled over onto his back and shielded his eyes from the gold seeping through the crack in the curtains.

"I guess so," I said.

We locked hands and laid there as if in a trance, familiar with that particular silence that entombed us, and the birds began to twitter as if the day was indeed dawning in paradise.

CHAPTER THIRTY-TWO

Confusion Corrected

Several hours later.
He said: "I won't sign this."

I looked as if I suddenly suffered whiplash right there in the chair I was sitting in.

"What do you mean you won't sign it, Helmut?" I said.

"Exactly what I just said," he said, his face unyielding.

"Jesus Christ," I said, leaning back, attempting unsuccessfully to contain myself. "You have to sign it! We both do!" I said leaning across the table and snatching the document from him and scribbling my name.

"Look! This is a part of the deal, Helmut," I said and slammed the pen down on top of the paper. "A part of the process Marc has to go through. There is no silver bullet to zoom us from here to healthy. They have to perform the catheter. They have to. Today. And I truly believe with all my heart that Marc will be fine – he's had this thing before – a couple of times even! And if, if, God forbid, something was to happen – he could be in no better place than here, but nothing is going to happen and it has to be done before the surgery. Plain and simple. So sign it."

No tic. No twitch.

The technician sitting with us intervened. "Mr. Mayer," he said, "this is really just standard procedure. We have to explain to the parents of our patients the risks associated with the catheterizations. And as I've said, the frequency of any complications is very, very low. And sometimes, not performing the procedure can put the patient at greater risk—"

"I don't want my son to have a blood transfusion."

"It is highly, highly unlikely that he will need a blood transfusion. Again, it is just my responsibility to explain to you the facts about any complications that may arise and one of those complications involves a risk of bleeding. Whenever the skin is entered there is a possibility of mild bleeding. Now, severe bleeding can occur, but just because it can, does not mean it necessarily will, but should the circumstance present itself, the situation can normally be controlled without much fanfare—"

"Fanfare means no big deal," I said.

"—and it is only in the unfortunate event that there is too much blood loss that a transfusion of blood would be required," the tech continued, "but this is hardly ever necessary. And besides that, our hospital has its own private donor program and all of our donors are subjected to great scrutiny. You can be rest assured that there is an extremely low risk of infection – if indeed at all."

With that, the technician sat forward on his chair, and studied Helmut who sat there mute. After a moment, the technician looked my way, and then slid the document from in front of me towards Helmut. He held a pen poised in his hand towards Helmut. It was Helmut's for the taking. Helmut didn't budge. I stared at him. He stared back at me. My heart beat like a kettledrum and his did too. We each could sense it in our eyes. Eyes that reflected all of what lie behind us and all that could lie ahead. I knew his position on the blood thing. The risk of infection was only a part of his issue. And I respected that. But now push had come to shove.

The minutes ticked by. And by. Felt like a lifetime. I literally had to bite my tongue to keep quiet because Bible truth lay in the fact that if I opened my mouth I would scream. I would scream indeed and probably look for something to throw. At him. Hard. Caged in by frustration I began to feel sorry for myself and got caught up in the warped idea of trying to imagine how it would feel to have absolutely no hope for salvation. To be helplessly stymied. It seemed like everything had gotten off to such a great start for us and now, this. The young man seated with us stood up and excused himself for a moment, unintentionally interrupting my 'Pitiful Pearl' moment.

Oftentimes, when it comes down to the nitty-gritty, resiliency is an extraordinary thing.

"If I have anything, I have hope, so bullshit on this little logjam. I've gritted this long, a couple more hours won't hurt," I said to myself. "I'll just create a calm center while I wait here because this is going to work out even if I have to sit at this table all day. Marc is going to have this surgery."

Helmut and I stared each other down, but finding the right ratio of hawks and doves was out of our reach. I knew that in Helmut's mind, the problem was not just a phobia of Marc getting someone else's blood. His parents had raised him in the Jehovah's Witness denomination and he strongly believed in their doctrine that blood transfusions were taboo. Though he was excommunicated as a young adult for not strictly following all of their rules and not confining himself to all of their restraints, he and Marc nonetheless had been having Bible study once a week for the past couple years in our home with Herr Klinger and his wife, who were members of this religion.

The connection was made because Herr Klinger and his wife were Helmut's customers. I thought it was a good thing for Marc to learn as much as possible about the Bible, especially with him being in the German public school system and receiving religious study only twice a week. I would have preferred him to attend a Catholic elementary school as I had, but none were available at the time.

The technician returned to a glaringly silent table.

"Mr. Mayer, I'm sorry," he said. "I know this is not an easy time for you or your wife," he added nodding my way, "but we've got to do something. The doctors are waiting and there are other scheduled appointments and—"

"I want to talk to Dr. Castañeda," Helmut said. My shoulders went slack and I dropped my head. In my mind, it was now a done deal.

An hour and a half later, Dr. Castañeda appeared inside the cath lab.

"Dr. Castañeda, I'm so glad you're here," I said rushing over to him. Helmut, right beside me said, "*Ja, ich auch, Vielen Dank.*" ("Yes, me too, thank you very much.")

"It's no problem," Dr. Castañeda said and then went on to basically reiterate in German what had already been explained to us by the technician.

Doctors Morrison and Keane began the catheterization at one forty that afternoon. They finished at two minutes past five. Marc lost thirty milliliters of blood. About an ounce.

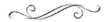

The Third Day.

We had previously been given permission, so early on Saturday we checked Marc out of the hospital for twenty-four hours believing that a 'change of wallpaper', as the Germans say, would do everybody some good. We spent the day getting a bit of cultural enrichment distracting ourselves from what was to come with trolley car rides, sightseeing and cuddling.

That night, Marc slept with Helmut and me in our room at the Inn.

The Fourth Day.

Sunday, we checked Marc back into his room at two o'clock. We watched television and played cards biding our time.

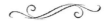

The Fifth Day.

At 6:30 Monday morning Helmut and I slipped into Marc's room. We let him sleep until 6:45, whereupon I woke him and helped him stumble through the fog of sleep to the bathroom to brush his teeth and wash up a bit.

"Mama, please go out for a minute. I have to go potty."

"Okay sweetie. Here. Mom will just walk you over to the toilet. I know you're still so sleepy. You call me when you're ready, okay?"

"Okay."

I left the room and closed the door. I could feel Helmut looking at me as if he'd lost something. I couldn't help him now. I stared at the floor steadying myself until Marc called.

I had just stepped back inside when Helmut popped his head inside the door.

"Guten Morgen, mein Sohn." ("Good morning, my son.")

"Morgen, Papa."

A moment passed and Helmut cleared his throat and said, "Are you okay, Marc?"

Marc nodded his head up and down as he continued brushing his teeth, eyes droopy with sleep. Helmut shut the door. A moment later, he cracked it open again. "Tracie, the nurse is here with the gurney."

"Okay," I said. "We're coming right away." I reached over to the door handle and pulled the door shut.

I wrung out the washcloth and gently dabbed at Marc's face. "Okay, little man. Ready?"

"Ja, Mama, I'm ready," he said sleepily.

I bent down, grabbed him and pulled him close. Felt his little heart beat against mine. I held him that way for a time, silently willing him with all my might to armor-proof his mind and spirit, his very essence to be unfearing and resolved to not take no for an answer and help Dr. Castañeda besiege this damned affliction. And come back to me and Helmut.

"Everything's going to be fine, my son. Hug Mommy tight. You're going to get some medicine to fall asleep and you won't feel a thing. And Papa and I will be waiting for you right next to your bed when you wake up. And when you do, you're going to feel so much better!" I could feel him nod his head up and down. I was sure the hammering behind my eyes would blind me. "God help me," I said to myself over and again. I sucked down stabs of terror with sheer self-restraint.

Magnificent self-restraint. Barely exhaled. It was all I could do just to hold on.

"I love you, Marc."

"I love you too, Mama." I kissed the top of his head again and again. "Okay, let's go, sweetie," I said.

The nurse helped him onto the bed and tucked him in.

"So, young man, now you can go back to sleep if you want to," she said to Marc.

Marc nodded his okay, but he didn't close his eyes.

"And Mr. And Mrs. Mayer, you can come with us down to the pre-op room and wait with him until Dr. Castañeda is ready for him."

Helmut's face flushed, as if he were fevered. We stood astride the bed, nodded our okays. Before we knew it, we had reached our destination. Four thousand some odd miles from home

It seemed a flashbulb illuminated the true-to-life snapshot with a single burst of light. A quick scan of silhouettes and symbols in the background; blurred images of doctors and nurses going businesslike about their work as they rustled by; a close-up of Helmut and me huddling over our son, teardrops on our tongues; and then Helmut holding Marc's hand as Marc is being rolled away until Helmut is forced to let go and then, as if in a time-lapsed frame, Marc turns and looks up to the nurse wheeling him.

He says something to her. Gradually, she slows the gurney to a halt. She steps to the left of Marc's head. Marc angles his head towards the right. He looks back at us with a smile. Raises his right hand, fisted, thumb up.

"That's right Mouse, everything will be fine Sweety!" I say with , 'Ain't no givin' up and no givin' out and 'Let go and let God' ringing in my ears and pounding in my heart as I stand there staring at him in awe, wondering at the amazing grace of Divine creation. Marc turns his head back around. The nurse sets the gurney once again in motion. The doors swing open and flap shut and the fading picture has merged Helmut and me into a single image clinging to each other in pain.

Canyon deep.

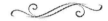

We were ushered to the family waiting room to wait during the surgery. It was half past seven. While we waited, Lisa, our surgical liaison nurse, had been coming in and out keeping us abreast of what was going on.

At 12:30 she informed us that Marc was being taken off the heart-lung machine and that a Fontan operation had been carried out.

She took a seat next to me. "It all went well," she said reaching over to Helmut and squeezing both of our hands.

"Come with me. Dr. Castañeda will be ready to speak with you shortly."

Dr. Castañeda sat down with us at a table in a small room and drew us two pictures: 1: confusion and 2: corrected. It had been white-knuckle surgery, but now Marc would be able to skip and run and fly and snorkel...he could live! A wave of faintness came over me. Pure disbelief. The next hours in intensive care would be crucial. We weren't out of the woods yet, but we were almost there. At last. After all this time.

And then that night, our dream turned into a nightmare.

CHAPTER THIRTY-THREE

The Saint and the Sinner

Tubes tunneled from various angles into Marc's body. He sucked fresh life into his lungs through an oxygen mask while lying dead flat, surrounded by specialized equipment. Cindy, his attending nurse that first day in intensive care, acknowledged Helmut and me with a smile, but never lost her pace, as she constantly moved around the bed pumping medicine into Marc.

Helmut and I cautiously approached the foot of his bed. Our eyes volleyed back and forth from Marc to the heart monitor. We each lightly rested a hand on either of his covered legs. He lay so still, but he was breathing. This was going to be a long night and once again I found myself contemplating the fact that sometimes what we are forced to swallow doesn't always easily digest.

With Cindy's guidance, we positioned ourselves so that we would not get in her way. After uncounted hours, she broke the concentrated silence.

"Mrs. Mayer, you and your husband should go down to the restaurant, get a bite to eat, try to relax a little. Marc is doing fine, doing just what we expect him to do. If anything should come up we will phone you right away, either in your room or in the restaurant, we have the numbers."

Helmut and I looked fleetingly at one other.

"But—" I started.

"I promise," she said, briefly patting my arm as she swept pass me. "Go, try and get some rest."

"Helmut, what do you think?" I said to Helmut.

"I'm not hungry," he said.

"Me either. Maybe we should just go get some fresh air for a minute. I'd like to change into some more comfortable shoes anyway."

"Yes, okay, that is a good idea." ·

"Cindy," I said. "We're going for a bit of fresh air. Just walk over to the hotel so I can change my shoes. We'll be back soon."

"Take your time," she said.

And so, Helmut and I clutched hands and reluctantly retreated from Marc's bedside and trudged over to our hotel room whereupon Helmut unlocked, opened and closed the door, and we each made a beeline across the room towards the bed and plopped down. We kicked off our shoes, fell back against the pillows, and just laid there staring at the ceiling. Holding hands. Supplicating silently.

Beyond the large-scale window before us, the protracted daylight of that May day was about to be forsaken for moonlight. Each minute that passed increased our hopes and fortified our optimism. Our fingers, so taut and so tired, little by little, began to unravel, releasing their entwined vise-like grip until our hands fell limp and loose, one upon the other.

And then a burst of ringing shot through the air.

Succumbing to an involuntary state of palsy that had been tremoring just beneath the surface of my skin, I leaped from the bed and seized the handset from the telephone. In my unsteadiness, its base went crashing to the floor and frantically I pulled at the spiraled cord, trying to hoist the swinging base back up onto the table without inadvertently pushing any buttons and losing the connection from the caller. Yelling "Hello? Hello?" just above the receiver cupped into the curve of my neck I could hear "Mrs. Mayer—"

I got things settled and gripped the receiver with both hands and shouted into the phone.

"Yes! Hello! What is it?! Is Marc okay? What's happened?! Wha—"

"Mrs. Mayer, Mrs. Mayer, it's alright. This is Cindy," she said. "I'm calling because Dr. Freed and his assisting attending doctors are here and have decided that it will be necessary to give Marc a blood transfusion."

I looked at my watch. It was shortly after nine P.M. "Why, what's happened?"

"*Was ist passiert?*" Helmut said, suddenly sitting upright. ("What's happened?")

"Just a minute Hel—"

"What's happened damnit!"

"This is Cindy and she says they think Marc needs a blood transfusion," I said avoiding his eyes, swinging around to reach for my sweater sprawled across the chair, stretching the telephone cord to the limit.

"What?!"

"Just a minute!" I said to him and then back into the telephone, "Yes. Yes. Okay. Cindy, look, please tell Doc—"

"Doctor Freed is here. He wants to speak with you. Hang on, for just a sec," she said.

A pause.

"What's happened?" Helmut said.

"I'm waiting for Dr. Freed to come on," I said.

"I don't want Marc to have a blood trans—" Helmut said.

"Sshh!" I said, wheeling away from him.

"I won't be quiet!" he said.

I spun back around and glared at him.

"Hello, Mrs. Mayer, this is Doctor Freed. Listen, I know how your husband will feel about this, but we're having a problem here—"

My throat constricted.

"We've tried various solutions, including giving Marc his own reserve of blood back which we promised your husband we would do, as well as giving him albumin to help carry his oxygen but nothing, unfortunately, is working. His hemocratic is way too low and I'm afraid if we don't give him the blood transfusion—"

"Dr. Freed says that if they don't give Marc the blood transfusion he's not going to make it," I said.

He had already swung his legs over the side of the bed and was putting his shoes on.

"Tell him we'll be there in five minutes," Helmut said.

"Dr. Freed, do what you have to do to save Ma—"

"Tell him we're on our way!" he said again.

Dr. Freed must have heard him shout. "Dr. Freed, Helmut and I are—"

"Yes, okay fine," he said.

I hastily put the receiver back in place knowing as I did so that a mutiny loomed on the moment.

I knew there would be no way to paint a pretty picture out of what I was about to tell him and even if there was, I did not have the wherewithal at the moment to convey it. There would be no stemming of his ire. So let him have at it.

"Helmut, look, if the doctors say Marc needs a blood transfusion, he's going to have to have it," I said. "Let's just be clear about it before we get there."

He grabbed his jacket and launched into his tirade. "You don't make the decision alone!"

"And neither do you!" I said.

"I don't want Marc to have a blood transfusion! You know how I feel about this and that is exactly the reason I spoke to the doctors about the information that Herr Klinger gave us about the alternatives and—"

"Look! Don't yell at me goddamnit! I didn't ask for it!" I said as I swirled about the room, grabbing my purse and searching for the room keys. "All that I'm trying to say is that if the doctors say he has to have one, then he has to have one! End of story! We really don't need to exhaust ourselves talking about it!"

"Tracie, who do you think you are to decide? We can't agree to it before we know that they've tried everything!"

"Marc's mother! And they did try everything! That's what Dr. Freed just said."

"Yeah sure! They tried everything! It's just easier to give—"

"What – do you think they're lying? Get serious! Let me tell you something, Helmut! I am fully aware about the information you got from Herr Klinger and I am fully aware that you discussed it with the doctors! I was there, remember? And don't get me wrong—I appreciate Herr Klinger's concern for Marc, and I believe in the Bible, and I believe in my heart that God can see my compassion and mercy and knows that I am not by nature a bad person, but if it makes me bad because I want to save my child's life by agreeing to a blood transfusion then I will be a bad person! And maybe I don't spread The Word from door to door, but neither do you – so who do you think YOU are trying to shove this down my throat?"

"It has nothing to do with going from door to door! How can you be so stupid? It has to do with what it says in the Bible dammit! And in the Bible it says that we should not accept foreign blood! And it's not just that! What about all the diseases that can be carried in the blood and the fact that each type has its own DNA and just like no two fingerprints are the same."

"First of all, let's get something straight right now. If I was so damn stupid it is highly unlikely that we would even be standing here having this conversation so don't insult me! Secondly, they already told us that the blood here is thoroughly screened and checked before Marc had the catheter! Remember? "Look, I said, trying to arrest myself, "I respect your beliefs."

"You don't respect anything! You just—"

"And I respect what it says in the Bible and I would rather Marc not have to have this just as much as you," I said, slipping back into a crescendo and my uncomfortable shoes, "but I am only human and if the doctors say there is nothing else to do then..."

"I will NOT let Marc have a blood transfusion! It doesn't come into question!"

I leaped up and threw my sweater towards his side of the bed, knocking a lamp over. "Why do I feel like I'm talking to a brick wall here? Everything is not always just black or white – sometimes there's a great big mass of gray out there, Helmut! And you might as well try to understand that your issue about blood transfusions being verboten is not the rule for me and I won't let it be the rule for Marc! Not as long as I'm breathing!"

He hurriedly straightened the lamp upright on the night table keeping his eyes fixed on me. We were both ungovernable now, revolting against each other and the situation at hand.

He gritted his teeth and looked at me. "You make me sick always thinking you are right with your let's do it now and rush-rush attitude without thinking something through! That is not the correct way to do things."

"The only time I didn't think something through was when I jumped up and left my family and my country and moved to Germany!"

"Well, why don't you go back?"

"If and when I do go back you won't have to worry about it and you can be damn sure that I'll do all I can to make sure Marc is healthy before I go!"

"I don't care what you say," he said. "I'm telling you that we can't and I WON'T decide to do this until I know they've done everything."

I started yanking at the hair on the sides of my head as if I'd temporarily gone berserk. "They have done everything! What is it about that that you can't or won't understand? I have the utmost faith in these doctors and this hospital! And the truth of the matter is you do too! They have respected our wishes and have done what was in their power to avoid this, but now it is the end of the road! We have no other choice! And probably not a helluva lot of time! Do you hear me?"

"Listen!" he said walking towards me. Spit balls formed at the corners of his mouth. His left hand whipped the air between us as he pointed at me in defiance, too close to my face. I'd never witnessed him rabid before. I stepped back.

And suddenly, I was in the office, watching Daddy shake his head the way he always shook it and say the two words he always said when he faced something downright unacceptable: 'No good,' I could hear him say. And then my voice welled up and I screamed the stars down.

"HELL NO! YOU LISTEN TO ME! This is our child we're talking about here! I didn't bring him all the way here and put him through all this just so he could die goddammit! That would be altogether stupid, now wouldn't it? Maybe I don't see the light enough to accept the Bible the way you do, but I know God loves me, Helmut, and I know He does not want Marc to die so I'll–"

"I don't want to hear it!" he said.

"Well, you're going to hear it! So I'll take the blame here! You be the saint and I'll be the sinner and as long as our son has a chance at a life," I said, rushing over to snatch my sweater from the bed, "I don't give a shit! I can really, honestly and truly live with that!"

I stormed into the bathroom, flicked the light switch on, grabbed a handful of tissues, switched the light off and stuffed the tissues in my purse. We both converged at the entry door to our room at the same time. I jerked the door open. Helmut slammed it shut.

Propelled by torrents of electricity, our mad dash over to the intensive care station was sullen and silent, each of us conversing with our own thoughts.

How I wished the deathlike gray pavement would veer off onto a yellow brick road towards some magical masterpiece of a destination where we would find a powerful wizard who would dazzle our eyes by revealing how to find a balance of forces in our relationships with each other and who would charm our hearts, increasing our capacity for spirituality and quench the thirst of our enquiring minds with universal answers to all of life's enigmas and who at the end of the day, would request our Maker to temper justice with mercy on our impeachable souls.

We could see Marc's chest heaving from the entrance doorway of the ICU. He hadn't been doing that when we'd left a little over a half hour ago. Dr. Castañeda had retired to his home for the day, but thankfully, someone had the quickness of mind to call him and just minutes after Helmut and I arrived, he was standing at our side.

Stiff with fear, I stared at Marc as I grasped what Dr. Castañeda was explaining to Helmut in German which boiled down to what Dr. Freed had already told me. It seemed as if it all took about one minute and before I knew it, what looked like an IV pole had been stationed next to Marc's bed and from it hung a bag, its claret contents compelled to bring about a quickening in our son. Within what seemed like seconds, Marc was breathing easy again.

I dialed the number to the intensive care station at two that morning. Marc had stabilized and was doing fine.

"What did they say?" Helmut said.

I switched the light back off and laid my head back down. "He's stabilized and fine."

"You know Tracie, I just want to tell you this."

We hadn't spoken since we'd left the room earlier. There was room enough for an army battalion to lie between us in the bed.

I rolled over, turning my back to him, inhaled and loudly sighed. He either ignored it or pretended not to hear it.

"You know there was no way that I would have let Marc die. It's just that I know that if I hadn't insisted that they save Marc's own blood and give it back to him and try to use other methods like the albumin or whatever you call it, it could have been that instead of Marc getting four units of blood – he might have needed twenty units, so even though I had to really, really work hard on myself to agree to this, this is a victory for me and a victory for Marc.

I...was...so...damn...tired. I felt like saying, "Well, Hoorah. Hoofreaking rah. Wear the laurels," Instead I said, "Let's just hope everything turns out alright in the end."

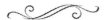

The Sixth Day.

Around three thirty that afternoon, Lisa, his nurse for this shift, took the respirator out and Marc breathed on his own.

"He's doing great!" she said. "He kind of had us a little nervous last night, but he's a fighter, aren't you, champ?" she said, leaning over our sleeping son and lightly stroking his hair. After a moment, she gave Helmut and me a wink and carried on with her checking, writing, controlling and adjusting.

Helmut and I stood on either side of the bed carefully touching and rubbing and kissing Marc who was there and not there.

"Marc, it's Mommy. Can you hear me?" I said leaning in close to his ear.

"*Und der Papa, Marc. Ich bin auch hier,*" Helmut said into his other ear. ("And Papa. I am also here.")

Marc's eyebrows arched as he tried unsuccessfully to draw up his eyelids.

He mouthed 'drink'.

"You want a drink? He wants a drink," I said glancing up at Helmut.

"He wants a drink," Helmut said back to me.

"Lisa –" we both said looking over at her near the foot of Marc's bed.

She'd heard us talking and simply nodded her tilted head in Marc's direction and smiled. He was deep asleep again. A while later he mouthed 'chips'. And then later: 'video'. On the video I told him he would have to wait and he grimaced in his sleep. Hah! Pleased as Punch about that piss-and-vinegar spirit!

As the day wore on, Helmut couldn't hide the very real trouble he was still having about the transfusion and to that end, he bared his soul to Lisa. I was just hanging on by a thread myself and knew that no matter what I would say to him, it would have been the wrong answer in his book. I felt like I was walking on thin ice every which way around me anyway and recall thinking that in a case like this, Daddy would probably say, 'sometimes baby, you got to know when to hold 'em and when to fold 'em.' Mama would say, 'just keep your mouth shut!' So that's what I did: folded 'em and kept my mouth shut.

Lisa, fortunately, really took his concerns to heart and in an attempt to assuage his distress, called one of the attending doctors to Marc's bedside whereupon they both explained to Helmut (and me) that they never let the hematocrit get so low. Ever. And after they finished speaking with us, they sent for Dr. Kerry from the blood donor department who came to visit us loaded down with forms and questionnaires and various other documents involved with the donor process for us to review and who further showered us with verbal information, explaining everything, very slowly, from A to Z on how the blood at Children's is screened and tested.

By the time he'd left, both of us had more of an ease of mind, undoubtedly me more so than Helmut, but that was okay, because I recognized that he would simply need time, which could be perhaps the fifth element after earth, air, fire and water of our being. Out of reach, uncontrollable, too much and never enough, indeed it is too often the most mangled thread in the fabric of our human existence.

Late that afternoon Dr. Castañeda stopped by. He put a hand on Helmut's back and said, "*Es geht Marc super! Es könnte nicht besser sein!*" ("Marc is doing great – things couldn't be better!")

Seventh Day.

Ten years ago today Helmut and I held hands on the front deck of my family home overlooking the lake and before one hundred or so family members and friends, swore to love each other forever. And we remembered that vow today, here with our son in the intensive care station. We held hands with each other and with our son whose tube from his nose extending to his stomach has been removed and who now has only an oxygen mask and two tubes in his chest and one in his ankle and one in his arm and who nonetheless shakes his head negatively to the question of 'do you have any pain?' and whose oxygen readings are in the low nineties – for the first time in his life. Helmut and I see how far we've come and we are both unashamedly moved to tears.

CHAPTER THIRTY-FOUR

He Ran

Eighth Day.

When Helmut and I walked into the intensive care station at nine fifteen that morning, we were not prepared for what we saw. Marc's bed had been elevated so that he was in more of an upright position, he was wide awake and on a tray before him was a breakfast of French toast, frosted flakes, cereal, milk, soup and a huggable Oshko teddy bear provided by the hospital. He enjoyed a couple bites from everything and shortly thereafter dozed back off to sleep.

Later that afternoon, lunch consisted of a chicken leg with thigh, crackers, chicken broth and celery sticks. The three of us played UNO, our favorite card game. Tonight Marc would be moved back to his own room whereupon one of my sisters would be there to surprise him. That was great, but the real deal was the Batman video, Aladdin watch, a new Game Boy with games and candies galore.

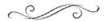

Ninth Day.

Marc walked today for the first time. It was a bit uncomfortable, but he kept at it and by and by, it got easier and easier. He seems to get stronger by the minute. Helmut and I strain, but cannot hear him gasping for breath. We walk dropped jawed beside him.

Tenth Day.

In the half light of daybreak, I noticed something different about me. I couldn't pinpoint at first just what this was. But I knew it was physical and I knew I couldn't see it. Maybe it will pass, I remember thinking.

The day was gorgeous. Marc and Helmut had breakfast and then I helped Marc dress, and the three of us went outside for another day of strolling in the hospital gardens. We clowned around and snapped pictures of each other in front of the bursting azaleas and even though the sign said 'Please Do Not Walk On The Lawn', Helmut wanted to snap Marc's picture in front of the fountain in its center and told him to "walk over there anyway." Hah! Walk over there!

We continued aimlessly along, stopping to play cards, napping, waking up and walking about at our leisure. As if it had always been this way. Eventually, we paused long enough for me, who never eats breakfast, to have a bite to eat. Marc and Helmut insisted they were still full from toast and coffee, eggs, cereal, milk, orange juice and everything under the umbrella of breakfast earlier that morning.

I settled on a real American tuna sandwich, thick with mayo and chopped onions and sweet pickles and lettuce on soft white bread, a cherry coke and a bag of Cheetos. I carefully unwrapped the cellophane from around my sandwich and slowly tore open the bag of Cheetos. I unfolded my paper napkin and laid it out flat on my lap. After flipping the tab open on my drink, all was in place. I bit into my sandwich and placed a Cheeto in my mouth at the same time. Chewed. Smiled and moaned in the affirmative; something like, 'Yes, Lord'. Popped in another Cheeto. Sat back. Chewed. Smiled. Swallowed.

"When was the last time I ate and drank this?" I asked myself. I took another swig of cherry coke 'til my heart raced and my eyes watered. I love cherry coke. Took another bite of sandwich and chip and sat back and tipped my chin towards the sun and closed my eyes and it was as if I was sitting amongst the gods feasting on ambrosia and nectar.

I swallowed and opened my mouth for another bite, but instead, I sat up and opened my eyes. Put my sandwich down. Helmut and Marc were paying no attention to me, which was good as this was a very private thing happening to me. Washing over me; a dawning. That thing I'd felt earlier this morning, that overwhelming sense of endangerment hemorrhaging through to my very core that I'd suffered since Marc was ten days old was ever so slowly abating. It still had me in its clutches, but it was now less intense, rather like smoldering embers instead of an out-of-control raging inferno.

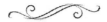

Eleventh Day.

Happy Mother's Day to me. Helmut was flying back home tomorrow, Marc and I had a couple more days to stay. Helmut and I took some time together and walked down to Dr. Castañeda's office to present him with an expression of our thanks, (if that were indeed at all possible), something we found in an antique store a few blocks away: a hand. Helmut and I were of one mind the moment we laid eyes on it. Larger than life, an intricately carved marble piece of stoneware, the extended fingers graceful and strong, the opened palm offering a nest of shelter and caring. A safe hand. As if it were tailor-made for Dr. Castañeda, this brilliant surgeon.

The sun was about to set on our last evening together as a family in Boston. Every minute had to count. Though Helmut's departure from Dr. Castañeda was a teary one for both of us, the real tears came when we got back down to Marc's room. Helmut stopped at one end of the hallway on our way there. He grabbed my arm.

"Sweetie, you go and get Marc," he said. "I want to wait here."

"Why? What's the matter?" I said.

"Nothing, just go do it," he said nudging me away. "Get Marc out of his room and stand at the doorway."

"Okay," I said walking away thinking that he must have a reason for telling me to do something like this, but didn't have a clue as to what it was.

A moment or two later Marc and I stood at the door of his room. Helmut stood at the far, far end of the hallway.

"Marc," he yelled, waving.

"Hey Papa! Was machts Du?" ("What are you doing?")

The nurses, at their station in the middle of the corridor, looked back and forth from Helmut to Marc.

"Marc!" Helmut said. "Run! Run to Papa!"

Marc looked up at me and smiled. I smiled back down at him. The nurses walked over to cheer Marc on.

"Okay Papa! Okay!"

He blew some air into his hands and then rubbed them together, looked up at me and winked. One of the nurses started to cry. I cried. And then Marc ran!

He ran!

He ran!

He ran!

THE BEGINNING

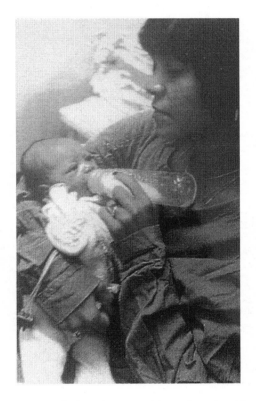

At the University of Cologne Clinic shortly after Marc's
birth

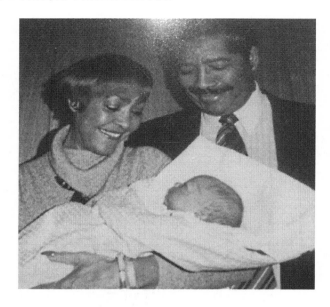

My mother and father holding Marc the day of his birth

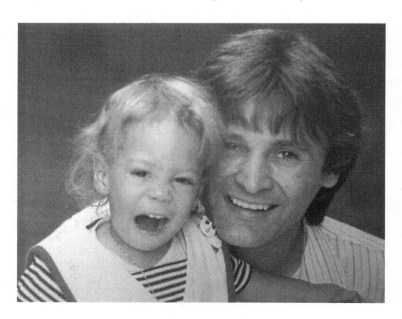

Marc and Helmut

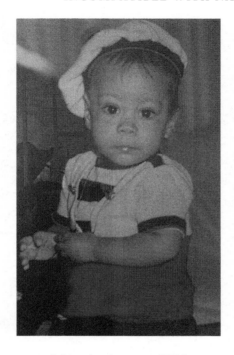

Marc in August 1986

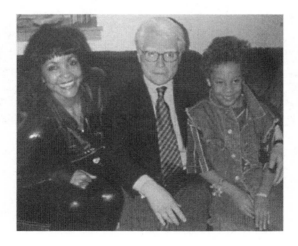

With Dr. Castañeda after Marc's surgery, Boston, 1994

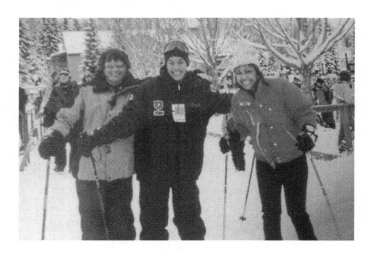

Skiing holiday 2003

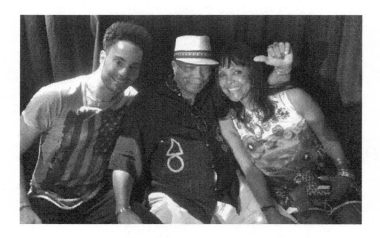

With Uncle Quincy Jones at the 2016 Montreux Jazz
Festival

And Now...

"To be able to help children born with a congenital heart malformation is very rewarding.

This story of Marc offers an example of how a determined mother never lost hope and how she pursued a worldwide search to provide the best possible options to save the life of her suffering child.

This is the personal history of a remarkable family and how they suffered through the initial news that their child was born with an extremely complex form of congenital heart defects and how they managed to live through two initial palliative shunt operations in Germany, followed later by a final operation by us at the Boston Children's Hospital.

After his complicated third operation, Marc is now a very impressive and accomplished young man. His family, in its dedication and commitment to their son's well-being, inspired me and I am certain will also move the reader of this well written, compassionate and compelling human story.

It was my privilege to know and to provide some help to this extraordinary family during their most difficult times."

~Aldo Castañeda, M.D. Ph.D.

As of this writing, Dr. Castañeda, at eighty-six years of age, is living in Guatemala City, Guatemala where he has founded UNICARP Hospital, the first pediatric cardiac surgical care unit in the country.

This center has become the regional referral base and source of training for physicians and nurses throughout the region and currently serves children from Guatemala, Honduras, El Salvador, Nicaragua, Belize, Haiti, and the Dominican Republic.

It is not unusual for Dr. Castañeda's team to repair the hearts of many babies and children of impoverished families at no charge. Dr. Castañeda has established *The Friends of Dr. Aldo Castañeda Foundation* to ensure sustainability of the program.

He goes to work every day.

If you can, please make a donation to his foundation. Make your check payable to *The Friends of Dr. Aldo Castañeda Foundation*. Mailing Address: Boston Children's Hospital, 300 Longwood Ave, Boston, MA 02115, United States.

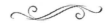

"It was a great honor for me to be for many years the pediatric cardiologist for Marc and his exceptional mother, Tracie.

The first meeting with her and her son was already unusual.

When Marc was born I was a resident on ward in the clinic for pediatric cardiology. One day the secretary of the chief of the clinic called me and said that a "blue baby", a patient of the chief of the department, was on the way to the ward.

The mother, Tracie, was a very good looking afro-American, dressed very colorfully like a pop star. And she didn't speak German. During the few following weeks, I found out that this "Pop Star" was an extraordinary powerful fighter, a fighter for the life of her son.

Marc had a heterotaxy-syndrom with complex heart failure including a single ventricle and pulmonary atresia.

In those days, the beginning of the eighties, dealing with these patients in Germany was controversial. It wasn't clear if it was possible to achieve a worthy life for them. The experience with the "Fontan" Operation as an ultimate palliation (connecting the systemic veins directly with the pulmonary artery bypassing the heart, today referred as TCPC = Total Cavo-Pulmonary Connection) was dull in Germany and the results weren't that good. So the family was advised by the chiefs of the pediatric cardiology and the heart surgery departments to let the child die peacefully rather than make him suffer all the many following surgeries with bad prognoses.

The doctors did their best to convince the family of this and it was assumed that Marc would quickly pass away. It didn't happen and Tracie started to rebel against the Gods in White. Against their opposition, she arranged for Marc to have the first palliative surgery at another clinic.

During the following years, many times over, Tracie had to put up resistance against the plans of different physicians, while she sought second and third opinions, focusing only on the best for Marc. Well, this may seem normal and self-evident, but everyone who is familiar with the doctor-patient interaction knows how difficult it is and how much power and courage it takes to disagree with eminent authorities.

Marc is now almost 32 years old, a great looking, strong and successful young man. And Tracie is a hero.

May many parents learn from her experience."

~Dr. med. Dipl. Psych. Alex Gillor

Dr. Gillor is still, after thirty years, practicing cardiology and working in cardiovascular research. His clinical trial validated the method of a non-invasive determination of oxygen saturation in the blood. He is a pioneer of this method.

To this day he remains to be one of my most favorite people. Ever.

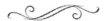

I am happy to share that Dr. Freed is now working part-time and enjoying his non-medical activities. I deeply express my gratitude to him for writing the Foreword to this story.

As far as I know, the Professor is still living in Cologne. I hope he is well.

Professor Maurice Bourgeois sadly passed away in June of 2006. He was seventy-two at the time and was deeply mourned by the medical community.

I never imagined that twenty-four years after Helmut and I pledged to be partners in life and love, and after all the uncharted terrain we'd successfully navigated together, that life would drive a wedge between us. The demise of our marriage had nothing to do with Marc or his health. It is, however, another amazing story.

That's all I will say about that...for now.

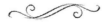

And from the mouth of my babe:

"Hey Mom,

Here are a few notes from me that I'd like you to share in your book.

The most important thing I'd like you to convey are my golden rules for staying strong:

1)   Believe in God.

2)   Trust your inner gut – you know your body, soul and spirit the best.

3)   Have a positive mindset – this helps the body to recover quicker.

4)   It seems as if people have lost sight of what really matters. Be grateful for your life. Stop looking at what you don't have and start being thankful for what you do have.

5)   Have a dream or a goal and stick to it. Everyone must have a dream, no matter how impossible it may seem to reach.

6)   Cherish your life, really cherish it.

7)   Time and life are precious. Nobody knows how much of it we have left, therefore we must make life worth living.

8)   Live in such a way, so that at the end you can talk about all the things you DID instead of about all the things you MISSED out on."

Marc received his college degree in business administration and has a career in the sales industry. After living and working in New York City, he has relocated back to Cologne – which thrills me.

Marc loves traveling, exploring foreign countries and their cultures like his mom, water sports, unlike his mom, and working out with me at the gym correcting my form and pushing me to the limit. ALL things soccer hover around the top of his favorite things in his life list and first place goes to as he says, "each and every day of my life being able to stay strong and healthy."

My kid.
My greatest achievement.
My pride and joy.

Grace and Gratitude

Firstly, I thank you God for your graciousness. You have been so very generous to my family and me.

To Vivien Theodore Thomas, cardiac surgery pioneer and teacher, Alfred Blalock, surgeon, Helen B. Taussig, cardiologist, Professor Francis Fontan, surgeon, and all of you brilliant cardiologists and surgeons who contribute to the world of pediatric and congenital heart surgery, this thank you is in recognition of your extreme aptitude, dedication and moral virtue.

To all of the doctors, nurses and medical staff who supported us, I thank you from the bottom of my heart.

To Uncle Boo, Auntie Audrey, Uncle Quincy, Uncle Lloyd, Aunt Gloria, Uncle Richard and Aunt Leslie, Auntie Margie and Uncle Chris, and Aunties Catherine and Janet, no matter where on earth I roam, you will always be that place I call home.

There are so many family members and friends who prayed for us, far too many to mention individually by name, but you all know who you are and I can never, ever, never thank you enough. I love you all, dearly.

Helmut Ehrhardt (www.multithread-solutions.com) as always, thank you for unfailingly being there for me, teaching me the rudimentary basics of how to use my laptop and repeatedly reminding me to relax.

A special thanks to each of the women in the Cologne, Germany group Writing Women. Your time and critiques were much appreciated. I thoroughly enjoyed sharing my heart with you.

Valerie Patton, thank you for asking me to join you on the trip to Vallarta. Love you Beans.

A tip of the hat to you, Lauren Logsted for your editing services.

A special shout-out to Deborah Woodson (www.deborahwoodson.com) for being my friend, understanding my issues, making me laugh out loud, and choosing the perfect picture for the cover of this book. Thank you Diva.

To my dearest friends Baaba and Chutes. You have been by my side since nearly the beginning. You are my family. I hope you know how much you mean to me.

To the Piano Girl, aka Robin Goldsby, (www.robingoldsby.com) you write first-rate novels, compose wonderful music, raise a beautiful family, can play the flute and the piano simultaneously and still have time to give me tips. You inspire me and I want you to know how much I appreciate you. You're the best.

Sharon Kae Reamer (www.sharonreamer.com) you are brilliant.

Your imagination, mastery of language and skills as a novelist are second to none. I cannot thank you enough

enough enough for holding my hand through this publishing process. I couldn't have done it without you.

Robin, my sister, thank you for coming to Boston.

Here's to all the days of making "quick runs" together to 106 and 165 and 319 and 324 and 419 and 509 and 718 and 901 and 924 and 1107 and and and...

Dana, my baby sister, when I left Seattle you were just on the cusp of womanhood. You have blossomed into a charming woman who is loved by many, but no one more than me. Your *joie de vivre* is at times wondrous and always contagious. When I think of doing the right thing, I think of you.

Delaneys forever.

Daddy, a standing ovation to you. There are moments when I deeply, deeply miss you. I cannot count the times when I find myself trying to figure it out, that I ask myself, what would Daddy do?

Wherever you are, I hope you're behaving yourself. Really. I mean it.

Mama. Mama. Mama.

You are tangible proof of love.

A bow of gratitude to you for showing me what it is to be a woman and mother. You and you alone are my inspiration in every single thing that I do. When I talk to myself, it is you who answers. Thank you for always believing in me.

Marc, I love you. That's a noun, a verb and everything in between.

A Woman's Story

Residing in Cologne, Germany since 1984, Tracie is a writer, lyricist, public speaker, real estate investor, and freelance English speaking coach. Please visit her website at www.traciemayer.com.

As an international businesswoman, Tracie is in demand as a bilingual moderator. Her most recent engagements include participating as jurist and moderator at the at the The ITB Berlin (International Tourism *Börse*) and as a guest speaker and charity fund raiser for the Austrian and German Children's Protective Agencies at the Vienna Filmball in Austria.

Among her many pursuits, Tracie supports various charitable organizations, including *Die Elterninitiative Herzkranker Kinder, Köln e.V.* (Parents Initiative for Children with Heart Disease of Cologne), the Ronald McDonald House in Cologne, the *Elternhilfe für Kinder mit Rett Syndrome in Deutschland* (parents' support group for children with Rett Syndrome), and the *Doctors for*

Ethiopia and the VITA e.V. Assistenzhunde (VITA Assistant Dogs Organization).

She is also an active member of the American International Women's Club of Cologne, a social organization with many philanthropic activities.

Together with her sister Dana, who resides in Seattle, Washington, she co-writes an upbeat blog. Visit them at www.menopausebarbees.com.

Tracie loves reading, the cinema, working out at the gym, and traveling. She maintains a girlish wonder and gratitude for the beauty she discovers in her various corners of the world.

She loves pink, but will wear any color.